Weigh
Fun a

sexy
Abs
Diet
POCKET GUIDE

By Alex A. Lluch
Health and Fitness Expert &
Author of Over 4 Million Books Sold!

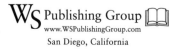

WS Publishing Group
www.WSPublishingGroup.com
San Diego, California

Sexy Abs Diet Pocket Guide
By Alex A. Lluch

Nutritional and fitness guidelines based on information provided by the United States Food and Drug Administration, Food and Nutrition Information Center, National Agricultural Library, Agricultural Research Service, and the U.S. Department of Agriculture.

For more best-selling titles by WS Publishing Group,
visit www.wspublishinggroup.com

Cover Photo:
iStockphoto/Stockphoto4u

Exercise Photos:
Nathaniel Kam, www.nathanielkamphotography.com

Model:
Anicka Pantano
ZARZAR Models
www.zarzarmodels.com

Meal Plan:
Lindsey Toth, MS, RD, www.lindseytoth.com
Image Credit: © iStockphoto/stdemi (fruit & vegetables)

ISBN: 978-1-613510-03-2
Printed in China

DISCLAIMER: The content in this book is provided for general informational purposes only and is not meant to substitute for advice provided by a medical professional. This information is not intended to diagnose or treat medical problems or substitute for appropriate medical care. If you are under the care of a physician and/or take medications for diabetes, heart disease, hypertension, or any other condition, consult your health care provider prior to initiation of any dietary program. Implementation of a dietary program may require alteration of your medication, which must be done by or under the direction of your physician. If you have or suspect that you have a medical problem, promptly contact your health care provider. Never disregard professional medical advice or delay in seeking it because of something you have read in this book.

WS Publishing Group, Inc. makes no claims whatsoever regarding the interpretation or utilization of any information contained herein and/or recorded by the user of this journal. If you utilize any information provided in this book, you do so at your own risk and you specifically waive any right to make any claim against the author and publisher, its officers, directors, employees, or representatives as the result of the use of such information. Consult your physician before making any changes in your diet or exercise.

contents

contents

Introduction

You know the frightening statistics by now: 67 percent of Americans are overweight and 34 percent are considered obese. Millions of people are struggling with their weight every day and suffering from the effects, from lack of energy to infertility to diabetes to heart disease, as well as the feelings of frustration and self-doubt that failing to lose weight bring. For many people, abdominal or "belly fat" is the most difficult to lose.

With the *Sexy Abs Diet Pocket Guide*, you'll learn how to combine diet and exercise in the most powerful fat-burning ways. This is important because belly fat is the most dangerous type of excess weight. A seven year study of more than 100,000 Americans found those with the highest waist circumferences have almost twice the risk of untimely death as those with the smallest waists. Interestingly, waist circumference is a significant predictor of mortality, even for people considered of normal weight for their height.

Belly fat is so dangerous because the cells are dynamic and active, pumping heart-clogging fatty acids into the bloodstream, creating insulin resistance, and sending hormones into overdrive (increasing risk of cancer). This type of fat is considered "visceral fat," or deep, hidden fat. High levels of visceral fat are found both in overweight people *and* inactive thin people. No matter what you weigh, a waistline larger than 35 inches for women and 40 inches for men indicates unhealthy amounts of visceral fat, according to the National Institutes of Health.

Healthy eating and exercise are the disease-fighting combination strong enough to lose belly fat and start feeling amazing. Neither will suffice on its own. You can lose 20 pounds and still not have defined abs. You can do hundreds of sit-ups a day and never get a flat stomach. Research has shown that *only* vigorous cardiovascular exercise can eliminate deep belly fat. A recent study that tracked the amount of visceral fat in three groups—one sedentary, one that exercised modestly, and one that exercised vigorously—found that only the group that got vigorous exercise saw a decrease in belly fat.

As you begin this book, you may have a hard time finding the motivation to lose the extra weight and belly fat. That's because so many diets are doomed to fail. They either force you to go cold turkey with the foods you love (causing cravings and bingeing), advise you to substitute real food with inefficient powdered drinks or meal replacement bars, or promote fast weight loss by eliminating whole food groups. These types of diets are neither healthy nor sustainable, meaning you'll only gain the weight right back. And you're not learning any new eating or exercise habits, so you'll simply revert back to your old unhealthy lifestyle.

The *Sexy Abs Diet Pocket Guide*, however, is full of the most powerful secrets to help you lose fat in record time. With a little dedication and some lifestyle changes, you can have the thin waist and flat abs you want. And you'll be healthier! Medical research has shown that losing just five to ten percent of body weight can significantly lower cholesterol and the risk of heart disease, stroke, and diabetes.

Losing inches and significant pounds won't be simple. As we age and our metabolisms slow down, it's tougher to lose the extra pounds. Your body needs a jump-start, just like a car with a stalled battery! You'll find the diet and fitness tips in this book to be just what you need to get moving, cook smarter, plan ahead, and eat better. And unlike other diets that eliminate the nutrients your body needs, you won't be starving or exhausted. The *Sexy Abs Diet Pocket Guide* contains a "flexible diet." You won't starve, eat only one kind of food, or miss out on dinners with friends—you just need to implement the diet and fitness secrets you'll learn in this pocket guide to lose stubborn belly fat!

Because your first step to a flat stomach and leaner shape is losing the extra pounds, the *Sexy Abs Diet Pocket Guide* includes three steps for weight loss.

1. Using a formula to determine the calories your body burns at rest, or your BMR.

2. Tracking everything you eat and all the physical activity you do daily for 30 days.

3. Creating a substantial daily calorie deficit—meaning that you are expending more calories than you consume through a combination of eating less and burning calories with exercise. The larger the calorie deficit you create each day, the more weight and inches you will lose.

At the end of each day, you'll total the calories you consumed. Then you'll subtract the calories burned from physical activity. Next, you'll subtract your BMR (the calories your body burns at rest) to find your daily total calorie deficit.

In addition to staying accountable for your exercise and your calorie-intake, you'll also learn to break bad habits that lead to stubborn belly fat, such as large portions, high calorie food addiction, and lack of sleep.

By purchasing this book, you have taken the first step in your weight-loss journey to looking and feeling amazing. In just 30 days, you'll be inches slimmer and sizes smaller!

How to Use This Book

Congratulations! You've taken the first step toward losing belly fat and cutting inches in a short amount of time. All the tools you need are right here! Simply eating less, making a few foods swaps, or spending some extra time at the gym isn't going to reduce inches from your waistline in 30 days. People who think they can lose considerable weight without any help get frustrated and fail. This book offers you many valuable features for burning body fat, getting in great shape, and successfully meeting your weight-loss goals.

Your personal health and fitness profile

Before you begin the *Sexy Abs Diet Pocket Guide*, you need to build Your Personal Profile. This section helps you assess your current physical state and fitness habits. With this information, you'll be able to determine your starting point, as well as identify your goals and any potential obstacles.

You will also determine the optimum amount of calories, fat, and carbs that you aim to consume every day.

Determining your BMR and creating a daily calorie deficit

An important part of the *Sexy Abs Diet Pocket Guide* is calculating your basal metabolic rate, or BMR. Your BMR is the number of calories your body would burn naturally, even if you didn't move all day. Knowing this number is the first step to this program, because building a calorie deficit sparks weight loss.

Every day, you will total the amount of calories you have eaten and subtract the calories you have burned from physical activity to find your Net Calorie Total. In order to lose weight, you need to create a substantial calorie deficit each day through a combination of diet and exercise. For example, one day, you may be able to cut 500 calories out of your diet, and then also burn 500 calories through exercise to create a 1,000-calorie deficit. Once you reach a 3,500-calorie deficit, you'll have lost one pound of body fat. Losing weight will cut the stubborn belly fat currently hiding your ab muscles!

Powerful diet secrets and tips, fast places to trim calories, motivational quotes, and more

Each chapter and section of this book is packed with the secrets of cutting calories, making lifestyle changes, and losing weight, because you can't get the toned, flat stomach you want without weight loss. Consider this: A University of Virginia study reported that to lose one pound of body fat you would have to do 250,000 sit-ups—or 100 sit-ups every day for seven years! Exercise alone won't give you a flat stomach and defined abs—it's the layer of body fat covering your muscles that needs to be whittled away through eating low-fat, low-calorie foods, and engaging in cardiovascular exercise in order to allow muscles to show.

With the *Sexy Abs Diet Pocket Guide*, you will learn to boost your metabolism, make healthier eating decisions, and develop a game plan for avoiding pitfalls as well as sticking to daily food goals. Through this book, you will practice conscious eating, curb your appetite, and stop sabotaging your weight-loss efforts. You will also learn to anticipate and recognize situations that cause you to binge or eat unhealthy foods.

You will recognize diet changes you can make without starving or depriving yourself, because no diet and fitness plan is going to work if you're feeling lethargic and hungry all the time. Burning hundreds of calories more than you eat in a day might sound difficult, but that's why this book is filled with "Did You Know" facts, motivational quotes, and quick and easy places to trim 100, 200, and 300 or more calories. You'll discover ways to lose weight that you never even thought of!

Eat from the customizable meal plan

The *Sexy Abs Diet Pocket Guide* meal plan lets you enjoy the foods you love, without the added fat or calories. Lindsey Toth, registered dietician and advisor to PepsiCo's Global Nutrition Communications department, has created a custom meal plan for this pocket guide that includes original breakfasts, lunches, and dinners that can be mixed and matched for smart eating throughout the day. Each meal contains a balance of carbohydrates, healthy fats, protein, and fiber to help you slim down, de-bloat, generate tons of energy, and feel satiated after each meal.

Eating from the meal plan means never having to guess about nutritional values, and makes recording your daily intake in your diet journal easy. Plus, the meals are simple and delicious, so anyone can follow the recipes and enjoy a well-balanced dish at every meal.

Ultimate fitness secrets for burning calories and body fat, and staying motivated

Fitness is the second key to losing weight and belly flab in 30 days. You can't do it with diet alone! The *Sexy Abs Diet Pocket Guide* gives you all the tips, tricks, and tools to maximize each and every workout and physical activity you perform. You'll get insight into everything from fitness basics to little-known secrets of getting in shape quickly without burning out.

In the Activities & Calories Burned chapter, you'll see that calories are burned in all sorts of ways, from sports to casual physical activity to normal household chores. This section is a great asset in finding sports and activities that you can incorporate into your daily routine to burn calories.

Powerful exercise program for maximum overall weight loss and core toning

The key to toned abs is to lose layers of belly fat and excess weight. The fitness section of this book includes a detailed exercise program that combines strength training with a cardio circuit six days a week to burn calories, tone the core, and cut through body fat quickly. Each day, you will alternate between a core, upper body, or lower body strength-training circuit. The last day of the week you will rest, recuperate, and relax.

Finally, the fitness section offers at-a-glance secrets for exercise and living an active, healthy life. The goal is to make physical activity a part of your everyday life—something you even look forward to. Refer to the secrets for getting fit in this section when you need a reminder of how to incorporate exercise and fitness into your routine.

Use your diet and fitness journal

People who keep a food and fitness journal are proven to lose *twice* as much weight as those who don't. As you read all the valuable, powerful weight-loss and fitness tips in this pocket guide, keep track of what you eat and drink in the journal in the back. Note the food and beverages you consume daily, as well as the physical activities you perform to burn calories. The journal enables you to easily see what you've eaten and to plan ahead for each meal and workout.

Keeping a diet journal will most likely be a reality check. Studies have shown that people tend to dramatically underestimate the number of calories in the foods they eat—by as much as 50 percent! The diet and fitness journal allows you to see your daily caloric intake, and to get real about exactly how many calories you're consuming. Once you recognize the high-calorie foods in your diet, you can replace them with lower calorie options, or reduce portion sizes. Additionally, recording your food intake keeps you accountable—because who wants to see hundreds of calories from a pizza-and-cheese-bread binge written in a journal? You'll think twice before indulging in a huge or highly caloric meal.

The journal will also help keep you motivated to exercise daily and provide a place to record your weight as the numbers on the scale begin to drop.

Your Personal Profile

Begin your program by gathering some information to assess your current physical state, habits, and preferences.

First, visit your primary care physician to have your cholesterol and blood pressure measured. These levels will affect the choices you make when creating your diet and fitness plan. You should also take your current measurements and a "Before" photo. It will motivate you when you look back and see a visual of where you began and how far you have come.

Next, assess your current dietary habits. Outline your goals, including the specific amounts of calories, fat, and carbs your diet should include on a daily basis.

Finally, reflect on your fitness history, including previous weight-loss attempts and obstacles encountered. Determine what you hope to accomplish with this program, as well as your overall fitness goals.

Your Health Profile

Request necessary information from your primary health care provider and complete this personal health profile.

Name: _____   Total Cholesterol: _____
Age: _____   HDL Cholesterol: _____
Height: _____   LDL Cholesterol: _____
BMI: _____   Blood Pressure: _____

Current Physical Activity: (sedentary, moderately active, very active)

_____

_____

_____

Current Diet & Eating Habits: (fast food, soda, snack often, late-night eating, etc.)

_____

_____

_____

_____

Other Current Habits: (smoking, drinking, lack of sleep, etc.)

_____

_____

_____

_____

_____

DATE: _____ **WEIGHT:** _____ **BODY FAT %:** _____

MEASUREMENTS:

chest:	biceps:	waist:	hips:	thighs:
_____	_____	_____	_____	_____

tape your photo here

PHOTO COMMENTS: _____

Dietary Habits Questionnaire

The following questions will assist you in developing your weight-loss program.

Which best describes your daily eating habits?
- ❏ Three average meals
- ❏ Graze frequently
- ❏ One large meal, little else

What types of food do you crave the most?
- ❏ Meat/fish
- ❏ Fruit/vegetables
- ❏ Bread/cereals/rice
- ❏ Sweets
- ❏ Salty snacks

Do you typically eat out or prepare food for yourself?
- ❏ I usually cook my food
- ❏ I eat out or have pre-made meals

What is your weight-loss goal?
- ❏ Lose 10 or more pounds
- ❏ Maintain weight
- ❏ Lose inches at the waistline
- ❏ Improve health

Which habits do you have?
- ❏ Skipping meals
- ❏ Emotional/stress eating
- ❏ Carb addiction
- ❏ Overeating while dining out

Describe your body type:
- ❏ Overweight
- ❏ Average
- ❏ Muscular

For what particular event (if any) do you want to lose weight?

_____

_____

What is your primary reason for wanting to lose weight?

_____

_____

_____

_____

Your Diet & Intake Goals

A huge part of your weight-loss journey will be managing your diet and intake. Record your goals and use them as a barometer for what you eat every day.

YOUR DIET GOALS

_____

_____

_____

_____

_____

_____

_____

YOUR INTAKE GOALS

Based on the number of calories your diet allows, consider the daily targets that you would like to meet. (Your primary care physician can also help you determine the appropriate amounts.)

Daily cal.:   Fat gms: Carb gms: Other:

NOTES: _____

_____

_____

_____

Your Fitness History

It is important to look back at your past experiences when trying to get into shape and lose weight to determine the diet and workout plan that will be the most successful for you.

Is there any reason why you should not engage in physical activity?

_____

At what age were you in your best physical shape?

_____

Have you ever participated in a workout program? If so, when?

_____

How long did you stay with the program?

_____

What did the program include?

_____

What inspired you to want to get into shape now?

_____

What obstacles have kept you from meeting your fitness goals?

_____

What will ensure these obstacles do not inhibit you now?

_____

Rate your current fitness level (scale of 1-10: 1=Worst 10=Best).

_____

Your Fitness Goals

By first identifying your goals, you can create a specific workout routine to help you achieve them. Your goals should be specific, quantifiable, realistic, and time-based. Answer the following questions honestly and objectively. You'll be able to use the resulting information to get inspired and avoid pitfalls.

What do you want to accomplish with this program?

- ❏ Improve cardiovascular fitness and endurance
- ❏ Improve diet and/or eating habits
- ❏ Improve flexibility
- ❏ Improve health
- ❏ Improve strength
- ❏ Improve muscle tone and shape
- ❏ Increase energy
- ❏ Lose weight
- ❏ Prevent injury and/or rehabilitate injury
- ❏ Train for a sports-specific event
- ❏ Reduce cholesterol
- ❏ Reduce blood pressure
- ❏ Reduce risk of disease
- ❏ Reduce stress
- ❏ Gain weight

What types of physical activity do you like and dislike?

_____

_____

_____

Do you prefer to exercise alone, with a partner, or in a group?

_____

Calculating Your BMR

Knowing your basal metabolic rate, or BMR, is crucial to the *Sexy Abs Diet Pocket Guide* program. Your BMR is the number of calories your body burns naturally at rest. Your BMR is based on your age, height, and current weight, and it decreases with age, meaning that it becomes harder to lose weight and keep it off as you get older. However, with a healthy diet and fitness plan, you can increase your BMR and lose weight more easily.

Use these formulas to calculate your BMR, then use this number in your daily diet and fitness journal pages.

Female BMR = 655 + (4.3 x weight in pounds) + (4.7 x height in inches) - (4.7 x age in years)

Male BMR = 66 + (6.3 x weight in pounds) + (12.9 x height in inches) - (6.8 x age in years)

Your BMR: _____

## Chapter 1

Changing the Way You Live

Losing weight and cutting inches takes a tremendous effort. If it were easy, everyone would be at their perfect weight and size. When you talk about a body and lifestyle makeover, you feel yourself getting excited, but when it comes time to actually implement the changes, your to-do list feels so long that you get overwhelmed and give up. Or, you make it a few weeks into a weight-loss plan, fail to see results, and quit. It's natural for the body to resist change. Your body tries to protect itself by slowing its basal metabolism, the rate at which you burn calories at rest, making weight loss difficult. However, the *Sexy Abs Diet Pocket Guide* will have you looking and feeling better immediately, starting with the simple lifestyle changes in this chapter. Read through them and commit yourself to implementing them. They are what your body and mind need to jump-start your weight loss, give you more energy, and get you motivated to complete this 30-day program.

Stay Motivated!
"Do not wait; the time will never
be 'just right.' Start where you stand, and
work with whatever tools you may have at your
command, and better tools will be found as
you go along."
~ Napoleon Hill

Mahatma Gandhi once said, "Be the change you want to see in the world." Being healthier and living better are goals everyone should strive for. You will likely find that after living the *Sexy Abs Diet Pocket Guide* program, you won't want to stop! You'll feel better and slimmer than ever before, and you won't want to fall back on the old habits that packed on the extra pounds.

Getting a flat stomach and sexy abs starts by modifying your daily routine. Today, you get a clean slate to erase the past and create a new, healthier, thinner way of living.

Keep your eye on the prize

Staying motivated is all about determining the top reasons you want and need to lose weight, and reminding yourself of them on the days you're tempted to eat a high-calorie dessert or skip the gym. Are you losing weight to look and feel great at a special event that's 30 days away, such as a high school reunion, wedding, vacation, or birthday? Did your doctor advise you that losing weight around the waistline will help reduce your risk of disease, lower your blood pressure, or help you get pregnant? Are you looking forward to the increased amount of energy you'll have after losing a few pounds? Or are you simply tired of feeling powerless around food? List the top three reasons you want to slim down. Hang this list where you can see it every day to remind you, along with a motivational image—a gorgeous beach, a dress you'd like to buy in a smaller size, the hike you plan to take when you have more energy, etc.

Create great new habits

Changing the way you live starts with building new, healthy habits that support your weight loss. One interesting difference between men and women when it comes to making lifestyle changes, is that men tend to zone in on a single task at a time, whereas women approach goals from a much broader perspective, often making it more difficult to accomplish every task. Think like a guy by tackling your biggest issues first, one at a time—be it that late-night eating, fried food, or overeating when dining out with friends.

Let's say you have the bad habit of overeating at lunch, leaving you sluggish all afternoon. Chances are, you're skipping breakfast (no, coffee is not breakfast), or eating empty carbs in the morning, such as a bagel or croissant. What you need, instead, is a protein and fiber-filled meal that jump-starts your metabolism and mind, and prevents overeating at lunch. Try having whole grains, such as wheat toast or instant oatmeal, with two hardboiled eggs and a piece of fruit or low-fat yogurt. Or, if you have more time in the morning, whip up a vegetable omelette with an English muffin on the side.

Get in the habit of keeping healthy breakfast ingredients in your kitchen or fridge at work, and you'll have made one awesome, positive change to your lifestyle. Focus on including each new behavior into your routine every day for a week until it becomes second nature.

> Did You Know?
> Depending on your height and body fat percentage, you could lose more than 10 pounds and as many as 3 clothing sizes in the next 30 days!

Eat from all six of the main food groups

There are six main food groups: grains, fruits, vegetables, dairy, meat and beans, and oils and sweets. Odds are, you've been overdoing it in some and avoiding others altogether. For instance, less than three and a half percent of American men and women eat the FDA-recommended amount of fruits and vegetables.

Unfortunately, when you omit food groups, you don't

receive the balance of protein, carbohydrates, and plant-based nutrients that your body needs. To kick-start a sluggish metabolism, maintain your energy, and inspire the body to burn fat cells, you must eat a balanced diet. The better you eat, the better your body works, and the faster you'll lose weight. You'll find it only takes a few days for your body to stop craving fatty and sugary processed foods. Some foods that pack mega-nutrients include low-fat yogurt, spinach, salmon, berries, avocados, whole grains, bell peppers, and olive oil.

Ransack your kitchen and pantry

Step 1: Get a big trash bag. **Step 2:** Open your cabinets, pantry, fridge, and yes, even the hidden spots where you stash treats. **Step 3:** Throw every high-calorie, high-fat, sugary, salty, processed piece of food into your trash bag. **Step 4:** Take one last look in the bag before you toss the bag into a dumpster. Say goodbye to unhealthy, bloat inducing, weight-inducing snacks and treats! **Step 5:** Feel inspired by your clean (perhaps nearly empty) cupboards and shelves. You now have a clean slate to start filling your kitchen with healthy foods. Remember, cravings can occur just by seeing these foods, so if you empty your cupboards, you can avoid them.

Break the addiction to high-calorie food!

Did you realize that constantly treating yourself to high-calorie foods can lead to an actual addiction? Eating a high-calorie meal triggers the release of dopamine and other feel-good chemicals in the brain. A 2009 Society for Neuroscience report shows that rats fed a high-calorie diet of bacon, sausage, and cheesecake had diminished responses in the pleasure centers of their brains over time. As the animals' brains reward circuits became less responsive, they continued to overeat and become increasingly obese. Their brains actually began to mimic those of rats addicted to drugs as they became addicted to high-calorie foods!

Break this cycle by eliminating these high-fat, high-calorie foods from your grocery list. If they're not in the house or in your desk, you won't be tempted. Don't even look at the dessert list at a restaurant. Simply imagining yourself eating a delicious crème brûlée can trigger an intense craving.

Get some shuteye

Research has proven that adults who get seven to nine hours of sleep a night eat less during the day and are much less likely to be overweight. When you're sleep-deprived, the body produces more of the hormone that causes hunger. Being exhausted also means you have less willpower to resist the temptation of fatty and sugary foods.

> Trim Up to 200 Calories!
> Pass: Croutons
> Swap: Pita for French bread on a sandwich

One study showed that lack of sleep can lead to eating an extra 900 calories a day. Wow!

Consider that cutting those 900 calories a day for a year would mean a weight loss of more than 90 pounds! To lose your belly flab in 30 days, you need to give your body the rest it needs. Try going to bed earlier and establishing a routine at night that is calming and gets you ready for deep sleep. For instance, surfing the web or watching TV can disrupt your ability to fall and stay asleep; instead, try reading for 30 minutes or taking a relaxing bath.

Bulk up your fiber and MUFAs at every meal

A high-fiber diet (25 daily grams for women and 38 for men) can help your body burn fat faster, especially stubborn belly fat. Additionally, by eating more fiber, you stay full longer, and eat less each day. Just be sure to drink lots of water as you increase your fiber intake to help your body flush waste.

You should also incorporate healthy monounsaturated fatty acids (MUFAs). MUFAs include oils, nuts and seeds, avocados, and olives. You should have some with every meal. MUFAs are your flat-belly secret weapons! They keep you full, and, unlike bad-for-you saturated fat, monounsaturated fats are flexible, and can easily move through your body without clogging your arteries or contributing to heart problems.

Add MUFAs to every meal. Cook stir-fry or make salad dressing with one tablespoon of oil; combine pine nuts and olive oil to make homemade pesto; add nuts or seeds to a salad; use up to two tablespoons of a nut spread on whole wheat toast; slice a quarter cup of fresh avocado onto a sandwich or alongside a lean protein; add sliced olives to pizza and sandwiches.

Back away from the TV

The National Weight Control Registry (NWCR) studies the behavioral and psychological factors that contribute to weight loss and its maintenance. The NWCR tracks more than 5,000 individuals over the age of 18 who have maintained at least a 30-pound weight loss for a year or longer (although the average registry member has lost an average of 66 pounds and kept it off for five and a half years). The NWCR has found that there are common threads among people who successfully lose weight. About 80 percent eat breakfast daily, and almost all maintain a low-calorie, low-fat diet, and high levels of activity. Additionally, 62 percent say they watch fewer than 10 hours of TV per week. By contrast, the average American watch 38 hours a week, almost four times that much.

Obviously, if you're spending numerous hours a day in front of the TV, you're not exercising. In addition, watching TV leads to eating unhealthy foods. Who curls up on the couch with a salad? As the NWCR study proves, getting off the couch and away from the TV aids in real weight loss. You'll eat less, and use the hours you spent watching sitcoms to hit the gym, go for a walk with a friend, or otherwise be active outdoors.

Drink little to no alcohol

Drinking alcohol makes losing belly fat tougher. Not only does the carbonation in beer and cocktails made with soda lead to serious bloating, your body processes alcohol first, before fat, protein, or carbs. Thus, alcohol slows down the fat-burning process. Also, a serving of alcohol contains at least 120 calories, and much more if you use sugary mixers. If you ingest 120 calories from alcohol, you'll have to either exercise more or eat less. That can be very difficult, since you're already going to be on a calorie-restricted diet.

Since the goal of the *Sexy Abs Diet Pocket Guide* is to find fast, easy ways to cut hundreds of calories, drinking alcohol is counterproductive. Plus, alcohol offers no nutrients, won't fill you up, and increases appetite, especially for fatty and salty foods.

Discover if you're lactose intolerant

To have a flat stomach, you must eliminate gas and bloating. This can come from the body's inability to digest lactose, a type of natural sugar found in milk and dairy products. Lactose intolerance is a common food allergy, and many people don't know they have it until they experience gas, gas pains, diarrhea, and other discomforts after eating dairy foods.

Lactose intolerance can be genetic and is more prevalent in people of Native American, Asian, African, and South American descent. If you think you may be lactose intolerant, observe the result of eliminating dairy for a week before reintroducing it. Your doctor can also confirm lactose intolerance with a hydrogen breath test.

To avoid bloating and gas from dairy, switch to soy or almond milk, and stick to dairy products naturally low in lactose, such as cottage cheese. Yogurt with live cultures may also be safe for people with lactose intolerance.

## Chapter 2

Maximizing Your Metabolism

We often hear about metabolism and its importance in helping us lose weight. But what exactly is your metabolism, and how can you make it work harder for you?

Metabolism is a series of chemical reactions that convert the food we eat into energy. This energy powers everything we do, from thinking to moving, healing, growing, and even aging. When you eat, you take in energy in the form of sugars (carbohydrates), proteins, and fats. But the body's cells cannot use energy in this form. The body breaks them down so the energy can be distributed to and used by our cells. Molecules in the digestive system called enzymes break down each substance differently: proteins become amino acids; fats become fatty acids; carbohydrates become simple sugars. The process of breaking these substances down and using them for energy is called "metabolism."

Metabolism is a complicated chemical sequence, so it's easier to think of it in its most basic sense—metabolism is a process that influences how easily you gain and lose weight, or how easily you store or burn calories. The number of calories you are able to burn in a day depends on how high or low your metabolism is. Earlier in this book, you calculated your basal metabolic rate, or BMR. This is the rate at which your body burns calories while at rest. Everyone has a different BMR, which is largely inherited. You have probably heard friends lament, "Oh, I have the slowest metabolism in the world," or "Have you seen how much so-and-so eats? He must have a super-fast metabolism." However, genetics don't determine everything when it comes to how quickly or slowly your body burns calories. You can actually change your BMR by engaging in certain activities and eating certain foods. For example, regular exercise can increase your body's BMR. Muscle burns three times as many calories as fat—about six calories per pound for muscle and only two calories per pound for fat. Therefore, every pound of muscle burns 30 to 50 extra calories per day. Finally, your eating habits—the times at which you eat and your intake of protein or other metabolism-friendly foods—can also increase your BMR.

Don't settle for a slow metabolism or use it to excuse losing weight. This chapter gives you tips and tricks to super-charge your metabolism, starting from the moment you wake up in the morning.

Eat breakfast

Breakfast is called "the most important meal of the day" for a reason, and eating breakfast is essential for weight loss. Your body is deprived of food during the night—you are literally taking a "break" to "fast." Consider that if you ate dinner the night before at 7 p.m., and you go all the way to lunch without eating, you'll have fasted for 17 hours or more! Your blood sugar will be extremely low. Plus, if your body doesn't receive sufficient nutrients post-fast, it will function less efficiently. Eating a balanced breakfast jump-starts your metabolism, helps you eat a normal portion at lunch, and provides blood-sugar stability that means more energy, brainpower, and focus for your day. A cup of coffee isn't breakfast! Whole grains, oats, peanut butter, fruit, low-fat yogurt, and eggs are all good ways to start your day. They get your metabolism kicking, and prevent overeating throughout the day.

Never skip meals

Dieters make the mistake of believing that skipping

meals will help them cut calories and lose weight. But when you skip a meal your system goes into starvation mode. Your metabolism slows to conserve energy, and your body prepares to store fat during your next meal. Additionally, too many hours between meals means you'll be so hungry you'll eat too much. Don't confuse your body by skipping meals; instead, eat small portions throughout the day. Try having three small meals and two or three healthy snacks. This keeps your metabolism working continuously and avoids blood sugar surges and crashes.

Eat small meals throughout the day

Increase your total calorie-burning capacity by having small, portion-controlled meals throughout the day. The act of eating helps increase your metabolism. The process of absorbing food requires energy. You burn calories with every meal as your body digests food. Keep your metabolism active by consuming small meals throughout the day. You will burn more calories while still eating the same amount of food.

Eat enough!

Ensure that you are eating enough to keep your metabolism active. Many people mistakenly believe that if they drastically reduce their caloric intake, for example to 1,000 calories a day, they'll be able to lose weight more quickly. However, your body and organs, such as the heart, kidneys, and liver, need a certain amount of calories simply to function, much less to fuel you through work, playing with your kids, and exercising. If you're trying to subsist on carrots, lettuce, and chicken soup, you'll be too exhausted to do much of anything but sit on the couch, and you'll never lose real weight. Find a healthy balance that lets you lose weight but provides enough energy as well.

Never go too long without eating

Waiting too long between meals can slow down the rate at which your body burns fat, as well as cause blood sugar dips that lead to overeating and feeling sluggish. Instead, try eating every three or four hours and choose nutritious foods—light cheese and whole grain crackers, small salads, hummus and vegetables, peanut butter on whole wheat toast, baked fish and chicken—and you won't overindulge at any one meal. Keep healthy snacks handy for those days when you're away from your office or house, and won't have time to fix something. You never want to go more than four hours without putting energizing food in your system.

Drink coffee and green tea

Coffee can be a helpful diet tool, as it suppresses hunger and kick-starts the metabolism. Research shows that green tea can actually help you burn fat and increase your metabolism. Green tea contains catechin polyphenols. These antioxidants help you drop pounds by increasing fat oxidation and thermogenesis, a process that increases body temperature as a result of burning fat. Green tea can also prevent storage of excess sugar and fat. Another antioxidant in green tea, epigallocatechin gallate (EGCG), has also proven effective at regulating glucose levels, which may reduce your appetite. Drinking five cups of green tea a day may burn 70 to 80 extra calories.

Stay hydrated!

Maintaining hydration is crucial for a flat belly and speedy metabolism. Water keeps your metabolism working hard, maintains digestion, improves muscle tone, and makes your stomach feel full. Water

Trim Up to 200 Calories!
Pass: Grande vanilla latte
Swap: Sashimi instead of sushi rolls

also aids in a flat belly by flushing out toxins, as well as preventing water retention (sounds counterintuitive, but true!) and constipation.

How much should you drink? You need to drink at least eight 8-ounce glasses a day. Men should strive for 120 ounces of water, and women should aim for 90 ounces. If you think about it, it's really not a lot. Fill a 750-ml aluminum water bottle (available at any store from Target to Starbucks to your local gym) three times, and you've already had more than eight glasses. Also try drinking a tall glass of water before every meal to help you eat less.

No matter what your ideal water consumption is, remember to increase water intake in conditions such as high heat, high altitude, low humidity, or during high activity. Water is necessary in order for metabolism to take place, so staying properly hydrated helps your body turn food into the energy you need for work, family, and exercise.

Eat spicy foods

Some research suggests that spicy foods, primarily red pepper, cayenne, and chili pepper, may help raise your metabolism. These foods may increase your calorie burning capacity for up to two to three hours after eating. The heat generated from capsaicin can increase your body temperature and temporarily raise your metabolic rate by eight percent. While studies need to prove whether or not this rate has a profound effect on weight loss, eating spicy foods may also help you lose weight by increasing feelings of satisfaction. The additional water needed to quench the heat they create certainly helps you feel full.

Add lean protein to your diet

Proteins are building blocks for your body. Unlike fat and carbohydrates, which are primarily sources of energy, proteins play an important role in the function and repair of body tissues. Proteins help build muscles, and can increase your metabolic rate. It takes more energy for your body to break down protein than it does carbs or fat because of the increased "thermic" effect of digesting protein. In all, the energy it takes to digest and absorb protein accounts for approximately 25 percent of the total calories protein contains. Ground turkey, skinless white meat poultry, as well as egg whites, fish, and legumes, are great sources of lean protein.

Eat "negative calorie" foods

Nutrient-rich, fiber-dense foods burn more calories than they contain. Even though fruits and vegetables have calories, they are referred to as "negative calorie" foods. Negative calorie foods usually contain high amounts of nutrients and fiber, and the high fiber content requires more energy to digest than the amount of calories in the food itself. Some negative calorie foods include asparagus, berries, broccoli, cucumbers, lettuce, grapefruit, oranges, melons, peaches, and plums.

## Chapter 3

Learning to Plan Ahead

Your life is packed with commitments that take time and energy, and this also makes it difficult to lose weight. If you're heading to an appointment around meal time, you will probably grab prepackaged or fast food, rather than making something fresh and healthy. And, after a long workday, pizza delivered to your house sounds much more appealing than cooking a nutritious meal. Or, you might skip the gym if a friend suggests meeting for drinks. Work, school, errands, family, friends, and other daily tasks constantly threaten to derail us from working out and eating well.

Unless you build specific healthy habits into your daily life, your intentions will fall by the wayside. In 400 B.C., Chinese philosopher Confucius wrote, "When it is obvious that the goals cannot be reached, don't adjust the goals, adjust the action steps." Sacrificing your health for your other commitments is not working. It's critical not to leave healthy eating to chance.

Planning ahead to avoid pitfalls makes the difference between cutting inches from your waistline and not losing any weight. Determine ahead of time what you will consume at each meal. Build a repertoire of healthy recipes and stock basic ingredients so you'll never be left wondering what to eat. Be prepared with healthy snacks. Treat plans to exercise as appointments that cannot be rescheduled.

Planning ahead reduces the stress of making healthy food and fitness choices, which can help whittle your waistline. Use the following principles to plan cooking, dining out, creating a calorie budget, and more.

Make a list of all the healthy foods you enjoy

Acknowledging that you'll need to create a calorie deficit, exercise, and avoid bloating foods each day for the next 30 days can feel overwhelming. Make planning meals and grocery shopping easier by writing a complete list of the healthy foods you enjoy. Once you list all the foods you love, you'll see you can still include some in your reduced-calorie diet, and your options will seem a lot broader and more appealing. For example, consider low-fat, low-sodium, and low-calorie dairy products, cereal, meat and seafood, soup and canned goods, frozen meals, salad dressings, prepackaged snacks, beverages, treats, and more, and make a list of your favorites.

Plan your meals for the entire week

Don't wait until Monday evening when your stomach is growling to decide what to cook for dinner. Use your weekend to plan your menu for the following week. If you plan ahead, you will be mentally prepared to eat smart. Also, you'll be less likely to overindulge on the weekend. Take a look at your schedule for the week and decide on a variety of tasty, healthy meals, based on the amount of time you'll have to cook. Then head to the store to purchase all the ingredients to prepare those meals. Make yourself a quick, healthy lunch option each morning before work—think salads with grilled chicken or salmon, or soup and half of a turkey sandwich with veggies. Preparing for the week ahead and making your own meals can save hundreds of calories per meal.

Know your "calorie budget" for each meal

Practice planning ahead by budgeting your calories at each meal. By recording everything you eat or drink in your journal in the back of this book, you'll know how many you have to spend to reach your daily intake goal. Consider any starters (soup or salad, perhaps), your main course, sides, and beverages. For example, have water: zero calories. Have a small side salad to start. Calories: 150. Have a 250-calorie turkey sandwich, hold the mayo, and you're at 400 calories. Now let's say you had budgeted 500 calories for this meal. You could spend that last 100 calories on a cookie, which provides a few moments of enjoyment, or you could save those last 100 calories. Save them, and you'll see the difference on the scale (and in the mirror) at the end of the week—guaranteed.

Have a game plan for dining out

A recent study showed that people consume 50 percent more calories, fat, and sodium when they eat out. But just because you're trying to lose weight and belly fat, doesn't mean you have to pass on dinner with friends—you just need to plan ahead so you don't overeat. According to Purdue University research, if you eat a handful of peanuts an hour before dinner, you'll eat fewer calories and less fat during your meal. Also, a broth-based soup or small side salad are good pre-meal choices. To eat less, anticipate what you're going to order so your eyes don't get bigger than your stomach when you're sitting at the table. Almost all restaurant menus are online now, and many also provide nutritional facts, so check ahead of time and decide what you're going to have. Consider ordering an appetizer, such as steamed mussels or a Caprese salad, as your meal. Restaurants are notorious for doubling and even tripling portion sizes. An appetizer or half-portion is probably all the food you need anyway.

Start a recipe folder

When deciding what to cook, you need an array of healthy options at your fingertips, or you'll be tempted to call for belly-bloating Chinese take-out or greasy fast food. Start keeping a recipe folder. Go online and print out healthy recipes from sites like CookingLight.com or EatingWell.com. Or buy magazines like *Real Simple* that offer fast, healthy recipes with complete calorie and fat information, and fill your folder with tear-outs. To flatten your belly, search for low-sodium or "blood-pressure friendly" recipes. You can also contact friends and family who are in good shape and ask for their healthy, tried-and-true recipes. Consider starting a healthy-recipe email chain that lots of people you know will benefit from.

Did You Know?
It's estimated that soft drinks make up between 5.5 and 7% of the calories in an American diet! If you haven't already, give up full-sugar soda immediately. However, simply drinking diet soda isn't enough. Remember that carbonated drinks cause the stomach to distend and bloat. And be sure you're not ordering the fried chicken just because you're having a zero-calorie soda.

Make a shopping list and stick to it

Trim Up to
200 Calories!

Pass: Butter on movie popcorn

Swap: Egg whites instead of whole eggs

Shop for only the items you need, and stick to the list you made earlier. Grocery stores stock the most tempting foods at eye level and in the center aisles. It's easy to get sidetracked if you let your eyes wander. It's also hard to resist a good bargain. Sale items can be difficult to pass up, so avoid the "end caps" of store aisles, which offer low prices on processed items that have a high profit margin for the store, like donuts, sugary cereal, soda, chips, and other unhealthy foods. You will be less susceptible to bright packaging, enticing deals, and other impulse items if you put on grocery shopping blinders and stick to your list.

Don't grocery shop when you're hungry

Stores use merchandising tricks such as product placement, overall store layout, and sale items to get you to buy more. These ploys encourage you to shop longer and spend more money. You may end up buying more food than you need, especially if you're hungry. Stop by the grocery store after a meal, when you won't be as likely to stray from your shopping list. Or drink a large glass of water. The feeling of fullness will make it easier to resist food. Also, chew a piece of peppermint gum while you shop. You'll be less likely to try free samples.

Plan ahead for travel

If you travel often and will spend a lot of time in airports and on planes in the next 30 days, you need a strategy that will enable you to continue losing weight. In-flight snacks are typically chips and crackers, with 200 or more empty calories in each tiny package. Airport food is even worse—pre-made sandwiches, personal pizzas, burritos, and barbecue are common layover fare, containing up to 800 calories and 1,000 mg or more of sodium. For early morning flights, bring packets of instant oatmeal and ask the flight attendant for hot water. Easy-to-pack snacks include raw, pre-cut veggies, an apple, dried fruits and nuts, and whole wheat crackers with natural peanut butter. For midday flights, make a sandwich (hold the mayo), wrap it in tin foil, and eat mid-flight. Other travelers will be jealous of your healthy, tasty meal!

Outsmart the minibar

Hotel minibars with salty and sweet snacks are very tempting to weary travelers. Practice this celebrity trick and save hundreds of calories by calling your hotel ahead of time and asking that the minibar be locked or emptied. It's too easy to give in to temptation when you're on-the-go, so plan ahead for an out-of-town stay. Bring healthy snacks with you, or stop by a grocery store to stock up on smart options to keep in your room.

Keep meal replacement options in your car or desk

There are times when a fresh, home-cooked meal isn't an option, so have some meal replacement bars and shakes on hand. While they aren't a long-term meal substitute, they are certainly a better choice than fast food when you need nutrition in a hurry. Stick to drinks and bars that provide a balanced 40/30/30 or 40/40/20 ratio of carbohydrates, fats, and proteins. Steer clear of bars with too many simple sugars, which add empty carbs, and don't satiate you over an extended period. Instead, look for a bar with more fiber, which will make you feel full longer. And stay away from anything that contains partially hydrogenated oils, or trans fats, which clog heart arteries.

Cook and freeze meals for later

While fresh is always better than frozen, many busy people enjoy the fact that frozen meals save them time. If you like the efficiency and convenience of frozen diet meals, try taking one evening or weekend afternoon to make a large batch of fresh food that can be divided into servings, frozen, and reheated later. Soup, chili, and vegetarian lasagna are just a few great options that can be made in healthy ways. Store each portion in an airtight container, freeze, and enjoy for up to three months. Having a frozen, pre-portioned meal on hand at all times means you won't be tempted to go for fast food when you're short on time.

Chapter 4

Curbing Your Appetite

Our need for food is first and foremost biological. Our bodies need calories, fat, nutrients, vitamins, carbohydrates, water, and proteins to carry out complex biochemical reactions that allow us to grow, heal, and function. But of course, if eating were primarily about giving our bodies energy, we would simply take a pill or gel that contained our daily nutritional values. In reality, eating is a social activity often dictated by our desires for certain kinds of food.

This love of food, or what we call "appetite," however, causes us to eat when we aren't hungry, to overeat a tasty treat, to crave foods that are bad for us, and to substitute eating for other activities when we're bored or restless. Our love of eating causes us to forget the primary biological reasons we are supposed to do it! This, combined with technological advances in food preparation and preservation, provides a dizzying array of choices through which to satisfy our hungry stomachs.

Controlling your appetite is one of the most important parts of losing weight and getting flat, toned abs. The best way to curb your appetite is to continually remind yourself that while eating is pleasurable, you should do so primarily because you have a physical need. Food is fuel for your day, for exercise, for mental focus, and for your well-being.

The tips and secrets you learn in this chapter will help you determine what causes you to eat when you're not hungry, restrict your desire for food when your body doesn't really need it, stave off cravings for high-calorie foods, and eat less overall to lose weight.

Identifying your hunger type

One key to losing weight is to identify your hunger type. People may eat when they're not hungry or overeat when they're extremely hungry and/or have low blood sugar. Sometimes people eat more in a social setting. Other times, they eat more sitting home alone, out of loneliness or boredom. One specific food may even trigger overeating.

Since you can't avoid food, you need to identify your hunger type and find a way to address that need in the right way. Determine if you're experiencing true physical hunger, low blood-sugar hunger, cravings, comfort eating, or social hunger. Once you're honest with yourself about why you're eating, you can put down the chips and wait until you feel true physical hunger to eat a healthy meal.

Know what foods trigger your appetite

Identify the foods that send your appetite out of control. These are foods that you find yourself compulsively overeating. Common trigger foods usually combine sugar and fat, or fat and salt. Binges are linked to the food itself; for example, if donuts are one of your trigger foods, a single bite can result in you eating three donuts, regardless of your hunger, situation, or emotional state. Until you're able to stop these impulses, you should avoid your trigger foods completely. Avoid even walking past the bakery section at the grocery store. Don't have a box of cookies at home if you know you won't stop at just one. For now, skip the office happy hour if you know you'll be tempted to binge on salty bar food.

Recognize that seeing foods you crave makes you want them more

Your sense of sight is a key factor in controlling your appetite and losing weight. Research has shown that

**Trim Up to
500 Calories!**

Pass: Frozen margarita

Swap: Yoplait Light
Red Velvet Cake
yogurt instead of
the real thing!

seeing and indulging in the bad foods you crave over and over actually forms neuron connections in the brain. Constantly activating these neurons reinforces them, and you begin to crave those foods all the time. When a person sees a favorite food, the brain becomes very active; even a photo of a tasty dish can increase your appetite. Don't linger over menus with images of high-calorie meals, and don't even look at the dessert tray. Don't let your gaze wander to other diners' plates when eating out. Simply recognizing that sight has a significant impact on your appetite will help you fight the temptation to eat when you are not hungry.

Steer clear of refined carbohydrates

Refined carbs are items made with sugars and white flour, such as white pasta, rice, bagels, donuts, and muffins. Ever notice how your morning bagel actually makes you feel hungrier after you eat it? That's because the body processes refined carbs so quickly that your blood sugar surges and drops. When blood sugar levels drop, the body feels hungry. So when you've eaten a 450-calorie bagel with cream cheese, you're ready to eat again mid-morning. Stick to complex carbohydrates that are low in fat and provide healthy protein, such as oatmeal, whole grain rice, yams, beans, and more. These foods slow both the digestion and the release of sugar into the bloodstream to keep levels stable and hunger at bay.

Alcohol may make you hungrier

A night of drinks and dinner may sound like a good time, but it will wreak havoc on your weight loss. The first issue is that liquids don't fill you up. In fact, research shows that alcohol not only decreases willpower, it whets the appetite and increases cravings for high-sodium, high-fat foods (consider traditional "bar food," like onion rings, burgers, nachos, and hot wings). As much as 20 percent more calories are consumed at meals when alcohol is served. Add the calories from the alcohol and there is a 33 percent increase. Secondly, the body breaks down alcohol first, before other nutrients, slowing the fat-burning process. The bottom line is, don't drink before or with meals, and you'll save hundreds of calories.

Slow down!

You eat quickly because of a hectic schedule, because you're on the go, or simply because you're a fast eater. However, studies show that people who eat quickly consistently overeat and tend to be more overweight than people who eat slowly. Also, eating quickly means gulping air with each bite, which causes bloating.

When you eat, your body releases hormones that indicate

> **Did You Know?**
> You may have heard that red wine is high in healthy-giving antioxidants; however, don't use that as an excuse for drinking alcohol and derailing your weight loss. Red wine contains 120 calories a glass or more, and alcohol is known to stoke the appetite. To benefit from antioxidants, try drinking green or black tea instead.

fullness and tell your brain that you are satisfied. It takes up to 20 minutes for this process to complete. During this time, it is very easy to stuff yourself with much more food than you really need if you're eating quickly. Use smaller utensils, take smaller bites, chew your food thoroughly, take a drink of water, and put your utensils down between bites. Try eating half of what's on your plate; wait 10 minutes, then have a few more bites if you're still hungry.

Go minty after meals

Studies report that mint flavor and smell may suppress appetite for a short period of time, so brush your teeth or chew a piece of mint gum after meals. The majority of what your brain perceives as taste is actually smell, so if you saturate your sense of smell with a strong odor, like mint, the smell of food will be less appealing, and you're less likely to eat more than you need. In one study from Wheeling Jesuit University, 40 people sniffed peppermint every two hours for five days, then sniffed a placebo for the next five days. During the week they smelled the peppermint, they consumed 1,800 fewer calories. Also, if you are susceptible to nighttime snacking, brush your teeth early so you won't be tempted to snack after dinner. If you can, keep a travel-sized toothbrush and toothpaste set with you in your car and at work.

Don't go cold turkey with cravings

Don't make your favorite foods off-limits, because you will immediately crave what you deny yourself. And remember—succumbing to cravings leads to overeating. When you eat sweet, salty, or high-calorie foods, your brain releases dopamine and other pleasure chemicals. When you deprive yourself of these foods, your body shifts into hedonism mode, demanding what makes it feel good. In addition, people have a tendency to want what they can't have, what is "forbidden." When you go cold turkey from your favorite foods, you dwell on thoughts of those more, until you give in to your craving and you binge. Instead, treat yourself, but in a smart way. Eat pre-portioned amounts of the treats you crave, such as the 100-calorie packs of cookies, crackers, and chips sold at all grocery stores. Everything from Reese's Peanut Butter Cups to Pringles now come in 100-calorie snack sizes. Allow yourself just one of these packages when the craving for something sweet or salty feels overwhelming.

Be the last person to start eating when dining out

People eat between 40 and 70 percent more food when in big groups. We tend to adopt the eating behaviors of the majority, no matter how unhealthy they may be. When you're in a group, be the last to start eating. Also, recognize that social interactions within groups tend to lengthen meal times. Longer meal times increase the likelihood that you will eat more. Don't feel the need to keep up with the table and match each bite of other people with your own.

Mix up your routine

Altering your routine can help you avoid the triggers and temptations that cause hunger and overeating. If you typically meet a friend for drinks and appetizers after work on Fridays, this may be a routine that has to change. Interestingly, the sights and smells of these familiar places may be enough to trigger your compulsion to eat. Meet your friend for coffee one morning instead, and order a flavored coffee without milk for a zero-calorie drink. Or, if driving past your neighborhood taco shop every day makes your stomach grumble thinking about mega-calorie burritos, take a different route. You can easily save 500 or more calories just by curbing that craving.

Chapter 5

Practicing Portion Control

A few years ago, the North American Association for the Study of Obesity performed a fascinating study on portion control and soup. Researchers gave some of the 54 participants a regular bowl containing a regular portion of soup, and asked them to eat as much of it as they liked. They gave other participants a self-refilling bowl of soup, with soup automatically piped into the bottom of the bowl as the participants were eating, making it impossible for them to ever reach the bottom. Researchers did not tell participants that extra soup was being added to their portion, and the soup was piped in so slowly it was impossible for them to tell.

Researchers found that participants who ate from the self-refilling bowl ate a whopping 73 percent more than participants who ate from a normal bowl. Perhaps more astonishing was the fact that those who ate from the self-refilling bowls did not report feeling any more full than those who ate from the regular bowls. Furthermore, the study found that a person's weight did not affect whether they were likely to keep eating from the self-refilling bowls. Participants eating from the self-refilling bowls included overweight, normal weight, and underweight participants. Across the board, everyone ate more, no matter the weight or mood.

This study proved what most people have already come to realize: The size of your portion determines how much you will eat, regardless of how hungry you are.

Another interesting study published in the *Journal of Consumer Research* in 2008, found that a concept called "extremeness aversion" also contributes to bad portion control, overeating, and obesity. Extremeness aversion is the tendency to avoid the smallest and largest sizes and ordering the middle one—no matter how large it is. According to Kathryn M. Sharpe, Richard Staelin, and Joel Huber, the authors of the study, this concept has gradually led retailers to offer larger portions. You may have noticed that movie theaters and fast food restaurants have begun to inflate the sizes of highly caloric items such as popcorn, fries, and soft drinks. The study showed that if a fast food restaurant originally offered 21-ounce, 16-ounce, and 12-ounce options for soft drinks, most consumers would choose the 16-ounce drink. However, when the restaurant eliminated the 12-ounce drink, consumers chose the 21-ounce, because the 16-ounce drink they preferred earlier was now the smallest size, making it less desirable.

Additionally, studies have proven that people are terribly inaccurate when it comes to eyeballing correct portions. A study referenced in the *Journal of Marketing Research* showed that consumers' perceptions of serving size can unknowingly vary as much as 20 percent. Another study reported that consumers vastly underestimate the caloric

Did You Know?

Don't fall into the trap of the "health halo," in which people consider foods labeled "organic," "fresh," or "low-fat" to be healthier than regular products. In a Cornell University Food and Brand Lab study, subjects were given organic cookies and chips, some labeled "organic" and some not. The subjects who ate the snacks labeled "organic" estimated the cookies had 40 percent fewer calories and thus, ate more.

content of the foods they eat. When researchers asked consumers to estimate the number of calories in various fast food meals, most participants estimated 700 to 800 calories—about half of the actual amount.

Portion control is three-fold: anticipating situations in which you may be served large portions; eating smaller portions; and feeling satiated by smaller portions. While this may not be easy at first, you'll quickly learn that you can be perfectly happy with less food. It should be fairly easy to recognize the environments in which you are likely to overeat. For example, certain restaurants are known for serving outlandish portions—two and three times the amount you need to eat. Or you may be aware that visiting family means larger meals. Having a plan for these situations can help you maintain proper portion control—and self-control.

Use these tips to keep your portions reasonable, and your weight loss on track. Controlling your portion sizes is one of the very best ways to flatten your belly and build a substantial calorie deficit every day.

Know the correct serving size for your favorite foods

Do you know a single serving size for your favorite foods, such as pasta, chicken, rice, or fruit? The reality of dieting is that you *can* eat most of the foods you love if you exercise portion control. First, that means educating yourself about what one serving really is!

Keep in mind that certain factors affect food portions, such as a person's age, gender, and activity level, but according to the USDA, one serving equals:

- 1 slice of whole grain bread
- 1/2 cup of cooked rice or pasta
- 1/2 cup of mashed potatoes
- 3-4 small crackers
- 1 small pancake or waffle
- 2 medium-sized cookies
- 1/2 cup cooked vegetables
- 1/2 cup tomato sauce
- 1 cup lettuce
- 1 small baked potato
- 1 medium apple
- 1/2 grapefruit or mango
- 1/2 cup berries
- 1/3 cup dried fruit or nuts
- 2 tbsps peanut butter
- 1 cup yogurt or milk
- 1 1/2 ounces of cheese
- 1/2 cup dry beans
- 1/2 cup tofu
- 1 chicken breast
- 1 medium pork chop
- 1/4 pound hamburger patty
- 1 tsp butter or margarine

Learn to eyeball portion sizes

There's no need for annoying measuring cups or a food scale—a handful here and a scoop there, that looked like a tablespoon, right? Wrong. Research shows that people can't eyeball portions without some practice. You won't always have a measuring cup on-hand, and who knows what an ounce of something looks like? Create a system in which you associate the size of a familiar object, like a golf ball or your fist, to serving sizes. After some time, you will be able to recognize correct portions just by how they fill up a plate, bowl, or pan. Here is a list to help you get started, or if you like, come up with your own serving-size associations:

- **Vegetables or fruit:** the size of your fist or a baseball
- **Pasta:** one handful
- **Meat, fish, or poultry:** a deck of cards or the size of your palm
- **Snacks (chips, pretzels, etc.):** a cupped handful
- **Apple:** a baseball
- **Potato:** a computer mouse
- **Bagel:** a hockey puck
- **Pancake:** a CD
- **Ice cream:** a tennis ball
- **Steamed rice:** a cupcake wrapper
- **Cheese:** size of your whole thumb
- **Dried fruit or nuts:** a golf ball or an egg
- **Cereal:** a fist
- **Dinner roll:** a bar of soap
- **Peanut butter:** a ping pong ball

- **Butter or margarine:** a postage stamp
- **Salad dressing:** a ping pong ball

Create a harmony between carbs, protein & veggies

A simple way to stick with moderate portions is to figure out the proportions of protein, carbs, and vegetables for your meal. Divide your plate into halves. Start by filling the first half of your plate with non-starchy vegetables, such as a salad, green beans, or grilled tomatoes. Fill a quarter of your plate with protein. Choose from fish, poultry, or lean cuts of beef. The other quarter should be a starchy vegetable or grain like sweet potatoes. Now you can ensure your meal is nutritionally balanced, and that you'll feel full and satisfied without becoming bloated or overeating.

Order single items rather than combo or meal deals

Fast food restaurants lure customers with combo meals that include a variety of items at a low price. Avoid these marketing ploys no matter how great the value. The amount of calories in a combo meal can contain more than a day's worth of calories. For example, a quarter-pound cheeseburger, large fries, and a 21-ounce milkshake have more than 1,800 calories. If you have to eat fast food, you can still lose weight by creating your own combo. Restaurants such as McDonald's will let you make substitutions, like apple slices for fries and grilled chicken for fried chicken. The kids' menu also often includes more reasonable portions.

Eat from smaller dishware and silverware

To help control portion size when you're eating at home, use smaller plates, bowls, glasses and silverware. Think about it: If you're using a large dinner plate, you're more inclined to fill it completely with spaghetti and meatballs—and then eat the entire plate of food. But if you eat with smaller dishware, it gives the impression that there is more food, so your brain will report that you're satisfied from a smaller portion. And using smaller spoons and forks means taking smaller bites, eating more slowly, and enjoying your meal longer, giving your body time to feel satiated.

Stock your freezer with healthy frozen foods

If your freezer is full of healthy frozen entrées as well as frozen meats and vegetables, you won't be tempted to call for take-out or get fast food when you're hungry. Stock up on meals with up to 400 calories, less than 10 grams of fat, and less than 500 mg of sodium, as well as frozen peas, broccoli, spinach, berries, boneless and skinless chicken breasts, fish, shrimp, pork loin, ground turkey, and more. On the other hand, items to leave out of your freezer include ice cream, alcohol, and any other temptations.

Use frozen diet dinner trays for portion control

Frozen diet meals are nutritionally balanced, portion-controlled, and provide an accurate count of how much fat, carbs, sodium, and calories you're eating. Another way to put your frozen dinners to work for weight loss is to save a few of the empty containers when you're done eating. Wash them out and use them as a model for proper portion sizes the next time you cook.

Don't put serving dishes on the table

Part of losing weight and exercising portion control is feeling satiated from a smaller amount of food. The sense of satiation is very visual. If you set bowls or pans of food on the table, you're simply encouraging yourself to take seconds. Serve yourself a reasonable portion size while you're in the kitchen, then put the rest of the food away for leftovers. This way you won't be tempted to take more of anything. Savor and appreciate each bite. After you eat, busy yourself with dishes and cleaning your cooking space—this gives your brain a chance to register that your body is full, and you won't feel the need to grab another roll or helping of potatoes.

Trim Up to
200 Calories!
Pass: Garlic bread or breadsticks
Swap: Spray salad dressing instead of bottled dressing

Take food out of its container

When you're eating out of a container, there is also a tendency to feel like you haven't eaten enough. If you take the food out of the packaging, your brain will register just how much you're eating. A yogurt may not look like much in its packaging, but you'll discover its contents actually fill a bowl. And how many times have you gotten to the bottom of a snack pack and commented, "There were only four cookies in there!" If you pour them out ahead of time, your brain has a chance to register that you are, in fact, eating a full handful of small cookies.

Order the smallest size meal when dining out

We all know that portion control is much easier when we're at home and can regulate how much we put on a plate. At a restaurant, portions are often two and even three times the size of what we'd serve ourselves. You must learn to identify a smart portion when dining out. Always opt for the smallest size available. Many restaurants offer a "bistro size" or "lunch portion" of their salads and entrées. This portion size should leave you happy and full. Or order an appetizer version of a full entrée, such a veggie quesadilla or steamed mussels. When you find yourself wondering, "Will the half salad be enough?" remember that restaurants often inflate meal sizes in order to charge more. Cut calories (and save money) by opting for the smaller portion.

Exercise nut portion control!

While studies have shown that people who include nuts in their diets often have lower risk of heart disease, nuts are also very high in calories from fat. Nuts are only beneficial if eaten in moderation, and don't significantly contribute to your daily calorie count. Unfortunately, because nuts come in large tins and bags, it's just too easy to snack on them by the handful, and wreak havoc on your weight loss.

Know that not all nuts are created equal! Good nuts include raw, unsalted almonds, walnuts, peanuts, and pistachios. Not-so-good nuts, such as macadamias, pecans, and Brazil nuts, are high in fat and calories. Because nuts are high in calories, stick to about an ounce, which equals 160 to 200 calories.

NutHealth.org lists the following as the number of nuts per serving:

- **Almonds:** 20-24
- **Cashews:** 16-18
- **Brazil nuts:** 6-8
- **Hazelnuts:** 18-20
- **Pecans:** 18-20 halves
- **Pistachios:** 45-47
- **Walnuts:** 8-11 halves

Nuts make an easy snack, just make sure you always count them out into snack-size baggies. Never try to ration while eating from a jar or bag—you'll overdo it. And be smart: Pass on anything honey-roasted, candied, or covered in chocolate or yogurt. Raw, unsalted, unroasted nuts are the ones that will make you feel full while keeping your calories and sodium down. In the right portions, they can be part of a successful weight-loss, anti-bloat plan.

Ask for a doggie bag right away

Another smart dieters' trick is to ask for a doggie bag as soon as your entrée is served. Determine an appropriate portion, and set the rest aside for leftovers. When the entire meal stays on your plate, you're tempted to keep eating until it's bare. Think about how many times you've thought, *Well, I've eaten two-thirds of this meal already, so I may as well finish the rest.* Store half your meal out of sight and feel content when the plate is empty.

Split your meal in half

You can cut calories and still enjoy your favorite foods by only eating half of your meal. Split your meal with a friend. Or, if you and your dining companion can't agree, substitute the other half with a broth-based soup, fresh veggies, or a piece of fruit. For instance, instead of two slices of pizza, replace the second piece with a garden salad and light dressing. This simple change can save you about 350 calories. Substitute water with lemon or sparkling water, like Perrier, instead of a soda, and you've saved 500 calories.

## Chapter 6

Choosing Healthy Alternatives

Americans tend to run in the other direction when they hear the word "healthy." Indeed, many people mistakenly believe that healthy foods are unsatisfying. In a new *Journal of Consumer Research* study, researchers told some students they were sampling a new protein, vitamin, and fiber-packed "health bar;" others were told it was a "chocolate bar that is very tasty and yummy, with a chocolate-raspberry core." When they were later asked to rate their hunger, students who sampled the "health bar" rated themselves hungrier than those who has eaten the identical "tasty" bar.

In a second portion of the study, researchers gave participants a piece of bread either described as being "low-fat and nutritious" or "tasty, with a thick crust and soft center." After sampling the bread, researchers offered participants pretzels; those who ate the "healthy" bread ate more pretzels than those who sampled the "tasty" bread. This study conveys that not only do people expect healthy food to be unsatisfying, it actually makes them feel hungrier. In the end, "healthy" foods made subjects eat in excess.

As a nation, we have been somewhat brainwashed to view reduced or low-fat foods as second-class to the original. But in many cases, reduced-fat or low-cal foods are indistinguishable from their higher calorie counterparts. Flattening your belly means you need to change your perception that healthy foods will not satisfy you as much as your favorite dishes. In fact, you'll probably find that once you continuously substitute vegetables, fruits, and whole grains for greasy, fried fast food, you will start to prefer the fresh, clean taste of healthy foods.

In order to lose weight and flatten your belly, you must make healthy trade-offs. Giving up desserts in favor of fruit, for instance, can help you drop unwanted pounds. Eating out less and cooking at home more saves hundreds of calories, grams of fat, and milligrams of sodium at each meal. In weight loss, trade-offs usually mean giving up something you enjoy for something less instantly gratifying, but healthier in the long run.

Nothing is more motivating than replacing bad habits with good ones, and seeing the unwanted pounds come off! Mark Twain once joked, "The only way to keep your health is to eat what you don't want, drink what you don't like, and do what you'd rather not." But this doesn't have to be true! Losing weight is really all about making smart trade-offs that have real benefits.

Modify recipes with healthy ingredient substitutions

There's no need to toss out your favorite recipes—just find healthy substitutions for high-calorie ingredients. Your favorite dishes will retain their flavor and save you hundreds of calories. You won't even notice the difference! A favorite diet secret is substituting Greek or other non-fat yogurt for sour cream and mayo. You won't lose any of the creaminess, but with zero grams of fat and tons of protein, yogurt is a smart trade-off. Tofu is also good substitute for many ingredients, because it is rich in high quality protein and contains no cholesterol. Try using it in place of cream in sauces. Replace ground beef with lean ground chicken or turkey. If a vegetable recipe calls for butter or margarine, use chicken broth and herbs for flavor without the fat. Replace whole eggs with two egg whites and just a tiny bit of yolk. Use condensed skim milk for whole milk. Replace the sugar in baking recipes with the no-calorie sweetener, stevia.

> **Did You Know?**
>
> Data from the National Health and Nutrition Examination Survey compared fruit and vegetable intake to USDA recommendations. Shockingly, less than 1% of adolescents, about 2% of men, and only 3.5% of women met guidelines for both fruits and vegetables—despite counting foods like jelly and orange juice as fruit, and both French fries and ketchup as vegetables. Eat more fruits and veggies!

Choose the right salad dressings

Salads can, of course, be one of your best weight-loss friends. Frequently eating green salads with raw veggies means your body will ingest crucial nutrients and antioxidants, such as vitamins A, C, and E, folic acid, fiber, lycopene, and beta-carotene. However, to slim down, you need to consider the dressings you're choosing. A Kraft Foods study of 1,000 people found that the top choices of salad dressing for women are Ranch, blue cheese, and vinaigrette. Men's top choices were Ranch, blue cheese, French/Catalina, and Thousand Island. Clearly both men and women favor creamy dressings. But they're the quickest way to sabotage your healthy meal. And beware of vinaigrettes loaded with sugar.

All salad dressings are full of calories, sodium, and fat. Instead, ask for oil and vinegar. A few splashes of balsamic or red wine vinegar are all you need, or squeeze a fresh lemon over your salad for a zero-calorie dressing. If you can't live without the Caesar or raspberry vinaigrette, try the spray bottle versions with only one calorie per spray (10 sprays are enough for a 1-cup salad). Don't turn your healthy salad into a 1,000-calorie nightmare; choose the right dressing.

Cook veggies the right way!

Never cook vegetables with butter, excessive oil, cream, or in the deep fryer. Instead, try a splash of lemon juice, a drizzle of balsamic vinegar, or a twist of black pepper before oven-baking vegetables, such as cauliflower or sweet potatoes. Omit the butter in recipes like curried carrots—the rich spices already give the carrots a great flavor without the added calories and saturated fat. Experiment and you'll find that many vegetables, such as tomatoes and bell peppers, are delicious when baked or blackened on a grill, without adding much of anything. Remember, the fewer ingredients the better when it comes to keeping vegetables low-fat and low-calorie.

Have whole fruits instead of juices

Whole fruits can help you lose weight because they contain essential phytonutrients, and their fiber and water content help you feel satisfied. On the flip side, commercial fruit juice usually includes added sugars and

100 or more calories per glass. Also, when the pulp and skin of the fruit is removed, the sugar absorbs quickly within the body, and can cause cravings later in the day. Juicing removes the bulk of the fruit, so juice does not fill you up. Half of a large grapefruit has 50 calories, two grams of fiber, and 11 grams of sugar, while eight fluid ounces of grapefruit juice contains about 100 calories and 22 grams of sugar. When you're craving something sweet and juicy, reach for whole fruit rather than sugary juice. For a dessert substitute, try putting pineapple slices or halved peaches on the grill for a warm, sweet treat without the high-fructose corn syrup and added calories.

Pass on prepackaged grocery store salads

When you're cutting calories, pass on prepackaged grocery store salads from the deli aisle. Typical choices— English pea, pasta, potato, Waldorf, macaroni, chicken, tuna, and egg salads—are all full of mayo. It's what holds these salads together and gives them their creamy consistency. These are not healthy sides. They are not "salads" like you want them to be—"salads" meaning fresh, healthy, and satisfying. A better choice that you can make on your own in a hurry is fruit salad. Chop a banana, apple, and red grapes, and add a can of drained mandarin oranges. Sprinkle cinnamon over the top and you have enough to feed two to four people a sweet side salad with no fat and only natural sugars. Another healthier, lighter option is to make tuna salad Mediterranean style, with chopped celery, olives, olive oil, lemon juice, and salt and pepper.

Enjoy a delicious bowl of soup

Warm liquids not only help relax the body, they provide a sense of satiation because they must be ingested slowly. Thus, reduced-salt vegetable soup is a great weight-loss food. Soup is relatively low in calories per serving, and the high water content sends messages to your brain that you're full. You'll have to slow down while eating the hot soup, and bites are always a spoonful. Have a tomato-based soup with high-fiber whole grains, beans, vegetables, and/or lean meat. If the bowl is small, pair it with a turkey sandwich on whole wheat bread (hold the mayo). The extra ingredients will take time to digest and leave you feeling full longer.

Avoid cream-based soups, since they contain butter and fat, and are high in calories. Also be sure to check the sodium content for soups, as some contain more than your maximum daily intake in one can! To avoid bloat and maintain a flat stomach, experiment with low-sodium soups, or make your own with low-sodium broth.

Incorporate veggies in unexpected ways

Fresh, fiber-filled produce is a big part of achieving a flat stomach; however, not everyone who wants to slim down also enjoys eating vegetables. Even people who love veggies typically don't eat enough of them! Rather than sitting down with a pile of produce and forcing yourself to eat it, try sneaking vegetables into dishes you already love. You won't even notice they're there, and you'll be getting the nutrients and fiber you need to lose weight and stay healthy. Some great ideas for incorporating vegetables in unexpected ways include puréeing carrots and zucchini in marinara sauce, meatballs, and burger patties; adding sweet potatoes to pancake batter; substituting baked butternut squash for pasta in mac 'n' cheese; and using steamed cauliflower in mashed potatoes. Vegetables are a crucial part of losing weight, because they are high in fiber but low in calories, so they fill you up longer. Plus, veggies are packed with natural minerals and vitamins to ward off illness and disease. Just because you're a former steak-and-potatoes type, or you're trying to cook for a family that refuses to eat vegetables, doesn't mean you can't get the nutrients your body needs to lose weight.

Satisfy a sweet tooth with spices

There are many ways you can satisfy a sweet tooth without cookies, cakes, candy, or ice cream. The urge for something sweet can often be satisfied when you add spices. Add the spices commonly found in desserts—vanilla, cinnamon, nutmeg, clove, ginger, and allspice—to other foods that are already naturally sweet, such as baked apples, pears, peaches, and sweet potatoes. You can achieve the flavors and sweetness you crave from baked goods without all the extra sugar, fat, and calories.

Find a low-calorie alternative to your daily latte

Unless you specify, coffee drinks are made with 2%

milk, which adds fat, calories, and carbs to your beverage. Additionally, any sweetener, such as flavored syrups, caramel, or cocoa powder, adds dozens of calories and carbs. And specialty drinks typically include whipped cream, chocolate shavings and other high-calorie toppings. Even if you opt for a light or "skinny" version of your favorite latte, you're looking at 150 calories or more.

> **Trim Up to 300 Calories!**
>
> **Pass:** Granola with raisins
>
> **Swap:** Turkey pepperoni instead of salami pepperoni

If you can't live without coffee, the key to losing weight is to pare down your selections. Start with hot or iced coffee. Sounds dull? It doesn't have to be! One or two pumps of sugar-free flavored syrup can jazz it up. A splash of nonfat milk is reasonable. Cinnamon is also a favorite coffee condiment of many dieters. It packs lots of flavor without the adding sugar. Making this switch will save 100 calories per medium coffee, a significant deficit, right from the start of your day.

Don't dip into fat and calories

Dips are popular at barbecues, potlucks, and parties, but most—spinach and artichoke, French onion, seven-layer bean dip—are packed with fat and calories. The most popular party dips are the creamy and cheesy versions, which have 200 calories or more, more than 10 grams of fat, and several grams of saturated fat. In addition, it's very easy to overeat when you're faced with a bowl of chips and a tub of creamy tip.

If you're attending or hosting a party, skip the veggie tray from the grocery store, which almost always includes Ranch dressing. Buy veggies individually (usually cheaper than the pre-made tray anyhow), such as grape tomatoes, celery sticks, bell peppers, cauliflower, and snap peas, and make your own healthy dip. A great option, even for the cooking-challenged, is hummus, which is just chickpeas, olive oil, tahini, lemon juice, garlic, and black and cayenne pepper blended to a smooth texture in a food processor. Or to make Mediterranean layered dip, a perfect substitute for high-calorie bean dip, you can stack low-fat Greek yogurt, kalamata olives, feta, tomatoes, red pepper, cucumbers, garlic, and whatever else you like. Top it with chopped romaine lettuce and a sprinkle of paprika for a healthy, hearty alternative.

Eat more natural peanut butter!

Natural peanut butter is a truly amazing diet food! It's a MUFA, full of heart-healthy monounsaturated fats, and the natural version doesn't include the hydrogenated oils, sweeteners, and extra salt of other peanut butters. You'll notice the label on natural peanut butter includes only two ingredients: peanuts and salt. It's a great food for flattening the belly because it maintains blood sugar levels and has fiber to keep you feeling full longer. Instead of a high-calorie muffin for breakfast, eat two tablespoons of peanut butter on whole wheat toast. And peanut butter on a banana or apple is a great snack. Although it might have as many calories as a bag of chips, not all calories are created equal. Peanut butter's fiber and healthy fats keep you full longer, so you'll eat less throughout the day.

Don't mess up the most important meal of the day

Yes, you need to eat breakfast—but it's what you eat that is either going to help you or keep you from dropping pounds. *Parade* magazine's annual report, "What America Really Eats," found that breakfast is actually becoming the highest calorie meal of the day for many people. That's because breakfast sandwiches and burritos—generally made with bacon, ham, cheese, fried potatoes, and eggs—made the top 10 on both men and women's lists of most-ordered menu items last year. Unfortunately, these items typically contain between 400 and 800 calories (not including the latte or orange juice you're probably washing them down with).

A better choice for shedding pounds and flattening the belly? Protein-packed eggs. A study from the Pennington Biomedical Research Center showed that participants who ate two eggs for breakfast lost 65 percent more weight than participants who ate a bagel, even though the bagel and the eggs contained an equal number of calories.

The egg-eaters also reported feeling more energetic than the participants who ate the bagels. Now, you do need some carbs, but make sure they're complex carbs such a whole wheat English muffin or oatmeal (without all the sugary toppings). Complex carbs make you feel full and burn directly into energy.

Beware of low-fat products

A report called "Can Low-Fat Nutrition Labels Lead to Obesity," published in the *Journal of Marketing Research*, offered insight as to why many people don't lose a single pound from eating low-fat or fat-free foods. The study found that both normal-weight and overweight participants ate more when presented with a low-fat option of a nutrient-poor and calorie-rich snack food. Additionally, they found that overweight participants were more inclined than normal-weight people to overindulge. Why? The study contends that low-fat food labels increase consumption because they decrease guilt and give the false perception that you can eat more of the item. And it seemed that this was particularly true for overweight subjects.

In a portion of this study, researchers set out two gallon-size bowls of M&Ms, one labeled "New Colors of Regular M&Ms," and the other labeled "New 'Low-Fat' M&Ms" (although no such low-fat product exists). As expected, participants ate more M&Ms (28.4 percent more!) when they were labeled low-fat. Furthermore, overweight participants took 16 percent more M&Ms

than normal-weight participants. While all participants increased their consumption, overweight subjects ate an average of 90 additional calories from the bowl labeled "low-fat."

Go easy on sugar-free products

Sugar alcohols found in artificially sweetened foods and drinks can lead to bloating and upset stomach, as the body struggles unsuccessfully to break them down. Low-carb or low-calorie products may be better for your waistline long-term, but to maintain a flat stomach, check product labels and cut back on anything that contains common sugar alcohols, including xylitol, maltitol, sorbitol, or erythritol, if they upset your stomach.

Know your bloat-free spices and seasonings

Do you salt your food at every meal? Are your favorite seasonings chili powder and hot sauce? You may be adding flavor to some foods, but you're also irritating the GI tract, retaining water, and causing the belly to distend. To look slim and slender around your midsection, learn what seasonings are salt-free and best for flattening the belly.

Ginger root, lemons, limes, and mint sprigs are all great fresh items that add flavor and depth to all kinds of food and beverages. Also, stock your pantry with fresh or dried bay leaves, basil, curry, paprika, cinnamon, oregano, Italian seasoning blends, rosemary, lemon pepper, thyme, tarragon, and dill. Mrs. Dash is another salt-free spice that's popular for spicing up chicken, fish, steak, and veggies.

Avoid cayenne pepper, chili powder, and hot sauce right before you're donning a swimsuit or form-fitting clothing if you want to show off your flat, sexy abs.

Deli meat goes low-sodium

Deli meat makes for easy lunches, and turkey or ham roll-ups with a bit of lettuce and mustard can be a great snack for slimming down. However, many types of deli meat contain high levels of sodium, and some even have dangerous nitrates and/or nitrites. Look for lower-sodium versions of your favorite brand of turkey, ham, and sliced chicken. Avoid high-sodium meats, such as salami, pepperoni, and bologna.

If you have time, the healthiest option is to cook your own turkey, pork, or chicken, and use the breast meat for sandwiches instead of buying sliced meat from the deli. To give you an idea of the difference, a 3-ounce serving of deli turkey can have more than 850 mg of sodium, while the same size serving of fresh, sliced turkey breast contains 75 mg.

Chapter 7

Exercising to Fight Fat

Too many people falsely believe they can lose weight by simply eating less or eating better, without sweating one bit. However, creating a calorie deficit from your diet alone, without combining diet with exercise, is nearly impossible, if not dangerous. In addition, an extremely low-calorie diet means you'll lack the energy and stamina you need to get through your day. On the flip side, many assume if they become moderately active, they can lose weight without giving up their indulgences of ice cream and burgers. Unfortunately, neither is a healthy approach and neither will allow you to reach your ideal weight.

Sit-ups alone won't get you a flat belly. A University of Virginia study reported that to lose one pound of body fat you would have to do 250,000 sit-ups—or 100 sit-ups every day for seven years. Before you can get a flat stomach and defined abs, the layer of fat covering your muscles needs to be whittled away through eating low-fat, low-calorie foods, and by engaging in full-body cardiovascular exercise, such as running, swimming, or power yoga.

Likewise, a Mayo Clinic report revealed the prevalence of "skinny overweight" people, or what is being called "normal weight obesity." As many as 30 million "thin" Americans are believed to have a body fat percentage and waist size that puts them in the overweight category and, therefore, at risk for disease, despite appearing to be of a normal weight.

Healthy eating and exercise are a powerful fat and disease-fighting combo, and only with the combination of the two can you drop unwanted pounds, get strong abs, and start feeling amazing.

Sexy Abs Diet Pocket Guide covers the importance of redefining your food choices, creating a game plan to address each meal and craving, and making healthy changes to your habits. This knowledge will help you eat hundreds of calories less a day and shed unwanted pounds; however, you can't lose weight, and keep it off, without exercise. You need to stay full and satisfied throughout the day. Cutting calories through diet restriction alone may very well mean you're eating too little, and eating too little leaves the door dangerously open for bingeing.

However, including exercise in your weight-loss program means you can easily reach a substantial calorie deficit without starving yourself. Just an hour of exercise a day burns hundreds of calories, making meeting your goal very doable. In addition, you will find that exercise is energizing, builds muscle tone, curbs your appetite, and increases your metabolism.

So what is the best exercise regimen for you? The answer depends on your personality, interests, and individual abilities. You can do it all at one time or integrate it into two or three segments over the course of your day. Just be sure to build a plan that fits into your daily calendar, and keep in mind that the common ingredient for any successful exercise program is to choose activities you will enjoy.

Incorporate all three elements of fitness

Your fitness program should include all three essential elements for successful weight loss and maintenance: cardiovascular activities to burn calories, benefit your heart, and reduce body fat; resistance or strength training for muscle tone; and a basic stretching routine to improve flexibility and prevent injury. Cardio is the most beneficial for weight loss and should be your main focus, but each element complements the others. Resistance and strength training will firm up muscles as the unwanted pounds melt away. Increased muscle mass will also burn extra calories throughout the day. Stretching and flexibility develop range of motion, increase muscle elasticity, achieve muscle balance, and protect the body from injury.

Trim Up to 500 Calories!

Pass: Tuna deli sub

Swap: Sparkling fruit-flavored water instead of champagne

When you perform cardio, you want to make sure you're moving continuously, and getting your heart rate up. You should be breathing hard. The rule of thumb is, be working hard enough during cardio that you can answer questions but not carry on a conversation. Typical activities include jogging/running, elliptical training, bicycling/spinning, and cardio classes such as step kickboxing, and aerobic dance. For strength training, aim for at least two 30-minute sessions per week that may include free weights, weight machines, resistance equipment, muscular endurance training, and toning activities such as power yoga or Pilates. Focus on activities that work each of the major muscle groups or work more than one muscle group at the same time. Stretching is important before, during, and after a workout. A study found that regular stretching can increase your strength by up to 19 percent when interspersed between weight-training exercises, for instance. Try doing 10 or 15 minutes of basic Ashtanga yoga poses.

Create a realistic schedule you can stick to

Schedule your workouts at the beginning of the week, when planning your meals. Be realistic! If you're not a morning person, don't schedule 6 a.m. runs. If you like to relax after work, don't pretend you're going to take a yoga class in the evenings. Plan workouts for at least five days a week, on days and times that are most doable. For instance, plan morning workouts for the days when you'll want to meet friends after work, or schedule a lunchtime hike for a day when you want to sleep in. Building exercise around your personal schedule and lifestyle means you're more likely to meet your goals.

Did You Know?
One of the best predictors of maintaining a fitness program over time is exercising in a social environment, like a gym or fitness class, or having a workout buddy. Think about it: The people you see each time you exercise become friends and acquaintances who expect to say hello to you, so you're less likely to skip a class or workout. Plus, you're making new friends while you slim down!

Get a walking workout

Many people starting out a fitness plan turn to good, old-fashioned walking. On a nice day, consider a stroll around your neighborhood. In cold or rainy weather, go to the mall and log miles while you window shop. Walking is a cost-effective activity that simply requires a good pair of shoes. Walking may sound too good to be true, but it is an aerobic activity that burns calories. Consider the fact that for a 150-pound person, walking at 2 mph, which is approximately a 30-minute mile, burns 189 calories per hour. Walking a 20-minute mile at a 3 mph pace uses 300 calories per hour. Walking a moderate, 15-minute mile, for an average of 4 mph, burns 300 calories per hour. The faster you walk, the more calories you will burn.

If you're not sure how far a mile is in your neighborhood, you can drive your car while looking at your odometer or buy a small pedometer to count your steps. The U.S. Surgeon General has recommended walking 30 minutes daily to strive toward a weekly goal of 10,000 steps, or roughly five miles. Those on a weight-loss program should strive for a minimum of 12,000 to 15,000 steps, which should take about 45 minutes per day.

Fend off food cravings with exercise

To increase your daily exercise and stave off cravings and hunger pangs, go for a walk the next time you feel like eating when it's not a snack or meal time. People often snack when they need a break from work or family, or when they're bored. Instead, try going for a 15-minute walk and letting the craving pass. Walking for 15 minutes will burn 75 calories for a 150-pound person. So, instead of eating a 150-calorie snack out of boredom, you'll have actually burned calories!

Find solutions to your exercise excuses

There are many excuses to skip exercise or to let a fitness plan fall by the wayside after a short time. But you won't be able to lose weight without exercise to complement a reduced-calorie diet. Write down the reasons you've been avoiding exercise, joining a gym, or taking a fitness class. Some of the most common reasons people use to avoid physical activity include:

"I don't have the time."
"I'm too tired and I don't feel like it."
"I'm not very good at exercising."
"It's not convenient to get to my workout place."
"I'm afraid and embarrassed."
"It's too expensive to join a gym."

Now write down solutions to these excuses. For example, if your number one reason for skipping exercise is "I don't have time," use half your lunch break to go for a brisk walk, or take a bike ride with your family instead of seeing a movie (you'll still spend time together and engage in something good for everyone's health). The bottom line is, there is never a good excuse to be sedentary. There are gyms and fitness facilities of all types and price ranges. If you find the traditional gym environment isn't for you, try a cycling club or dance class. If money is a concern, sign up for a hiking club—hiking, swimming, and rollerblading are always free. There are hundreds of ways to burn calories, so stop making excuses—make time and find something you like to do.

Take measures to avoid injury

Nothing puts a cramp in your weight loss like an injury. And if it's serious, it can mean the end of your exercise plan altogether. There are several ways to avoid injury when you're embarking on a new fitness plan. Always warm up and cool down for at least five to ten minutes before and after workouts. This is especially important if you're doing early morning cardio, because your body will be completely cold—like giving a car a chance to warm up. Also, give your body time to rest in between workouts. Get in a few hard workouts, but take one day off each week. For strength training, take at least one day off between sessions that work the same muscle group, so you give the muscle fibers time to heal and strengthen. Finally, be sure you ask a trainer the proper form and technique for exercises and machines that are new to you to avoid pulling or straining a muscle.

Use your fitness journal!

In order to slim down and get the abs you want in just 30 days, you need to expend more calories per day than you eat. Therefore, exercise must become part of your routine. The best way to see your progress and maintain motivation is to keep track of the days you exercise in the 30-day journal in the back of this book. Seeing the days accumulate on your calendar will really keep you motivated for the times when the gym sounds less than tempting. Write down the activity you performed and the duration of time. Keep track of everything you do, and don't underestimate what may seem like an insignificant activity, such as walking your dog. Consider that a 150-pound person will burn 100 calories from just a 20-minute walk at a moderate pace. Every little bit counts, just like with calories, so write it down and applaud yourself for making time throughout the day to get moving.

Join an online weight-loss community

Create a profile page at an online weight-loss and fitness community, and you'll have instant access to a huge group of people with similar goals, questions, obstacles, and tips for success. Seeing what works for others gives you motivation, and hearing about the ups and downs of exercise and losing weight from real people provides comfort and a sense of solidarity.

Enlist a virtual trainer

Hiring a personal trainer can be a great motivator and learning experience, but not everyone is ready for the time or money commitment it requires. A terrific option is a virtual trainer. A real person will create a fitness plan specifically for you, based on your goals and the equipment you have available. You'll get online tutorials on the proper form for exercises, worksheets for tracking progress, as well as reminders and check-ins.

Never give up!

"Don't give up, don't ever give up," legendary college basketball coach Jim Valvano told the crowd at the 1993 ESPY Awards, a night celebrating the accomplishments of the greatest athletes in the world. Inspired by Valvano's fight against bone cancer, the athletes in the room also knew plenty about the resilience it takes to stay in top shape. Valvano's words should inspire you too!

Losing weight takes determination and resilience. If you have a busy day, it's tempting to spend an evening on the couch instead of going for a run or bike ride. It's also tough to return to an exercise schedule if you've missed a few days. But don't decide you've failed. If you skip a day of your workout, tell yourself you'll start again tomorrow. If you overindulge at a meal, be firm that you'll have a longer, tougher workout the next day. If you feel like skipping the gym, tell yourself you'll do 30 minutes (odds are, you'll stay longer). Don't give up!

## Chapter 8

Maximizing Your Workouts

To lose stubborn belly flab and weight, you need to make the most of every workout or physical activity. You don't want to do the same exercises or routine every day for 30 days. To optimize the amount of calories and body fat you burn during each workout and lose as much weight as you can, use the tips and tricks in this chapter to learn when and how to work out, how to dress for your chosen activity, and how to stay motivated on days when you're feeling sluggish or lazy.

There is a lot to remember when starting an intense fitness program like this one. In this chapter, you'll learn the amount of weight you should be lifting during strength training, how to calculate your maximum and target heart rates, find how much water you should be drinking, and determine the best time to get new shoes.

Use the tips, formulas, and principles of fitness in this chapter to maximize your workout results. Nothing will make you feel better or more excited to maintain your program. With 30 days to go, you have no time to waste!

Work the "afterburn"

Perform cardiovascular exercise first thing in the morning! During the night, your body becomes depleted of your primary energy source, carbohydrates. Your body then begins to work from its secondary source, which is fat. During a pre-breakfast morning workout, the body will burn more fat. You'll also have what is called the "afterburn effect," which means the metabolism stays elevated for several hours after your workout. Finally, morning workouts give you an endorphin rush. This natural high can last for hours—even better than coffee!

Lift the right amount of weight

Building muscle helps you lose fat and drop unwanted pounds, but do you know the right amount of weight to lift during strength training? If you lift weights that are too light, you won't see improvements in strength or muscle tone. If you lift weights that are too heavy, you'll compromise form, and risk getting injured. You want to be able to perform eight to 12 repetitions per set, choosing weights heavy enough that you struggle through your final few reps, but not so heavy that you sacrifice form. You should be maxed out by the last rep; if you feel like you could do another, increase the weight by five to ten percent.

Another way to determine the weight you should be lifting is to find your "one rep max" for an exercise (the weight at which you can only do one rep), then lift 60 to 80 percent of that amount.

Know how and when to eat to maximize your workouts

It's important to know which foods to eat before and after you exercise. Carbs that are low in fat give you the energy you need to have a great workout. Protein helps with muscle repair and growth. Good fats also act as fuel for workouts, although you should eat mostly unsaturated fats, such as those from nuts, avocados, and fish.

Give yourself plenty of time for your body to digest before working out, and specifically avoid fatty foods before exercising. Fats remain in your stomach longer, causing you to feel uncomfortable. However, having low blood sugar before a workout can cause dizziness and lethargy, so if you're famished, a small snack of peanut butter or low-fat cheese on whole wheat crackers can give you the boost you need to make it through an exercise session. After your workout, eating a meal packed with protein and carbohydrates within two hours can help replace energy-fueling glycogen stores.

Include interval training to torch calories and body fat

Your mission is to reduce your caloric intake or burn more calories through exercise than you take in a day. Interval training is a great way to blast through calories and body fat because it combines short bursts of intense activity with periods of lighter activity. As your cardiovascular fitness improves, you'll be able to go longer and increase the intensity of the more difficult portions, helping you burn even more calories.

Here is one interval training workout that burns 500 or more calories in an hour on a treadmill. Eventually, aim for a sprinting pace of at least 7.5 mph, a running pace of at least 6 mph, and a jogging pace of at least 5 mph.

Begin at 0:00 on the treadmill and use the following 60-minute plan.

Interval training workout:

00:00–10:00	Warm up jog
10:00–10:20	Sprint
10:20–11:20	Jog
11:20–11:40	Sprint
11:40–12:40	Jog
12:40–13:00	Sprint
13:00–17:00	Jog
17:00–27:00	Run
27:00–31:00	Jog
31:00–35:00	Run
35:00–39:00	Jog
39:00–43:00	Run
43:00–47:00	Jog
47:00–51:00	Run
51:00–55:00	Jog
55:00–60:00	Gradually slow pace to jog/ walk to cool down

Wear the right shoes

Having the right footwear improves your workout. Wearing the appropriate shoes for the activity also protects you from soreness and injury. For instance, running shoes are designed for forward heel-to-toe motion, and do not provide the right ankle support for the side-to-side motion of activities like kickboxing or step aerobics. And depending on whether you supinate (run on the outside of your feet) or overpronate (your feet roll inward as you run), you'll need different types of running shoes. If you check out your old shoes, you should be able to see where the heel is worn down. Or visit a specialty store to have your shoes professionally fit. A shoe should be snug but not so tight that it puts pressure on the top of your foot or crushes your toes. And be sure to replace shoes every 300 to 500 miles.

Stay hydrated

Proper hydration is one of the easiest and most effective ways of boosting workout performance. Water is necessary for metabolism to take place, so being properly hydrated helps your body turn food into the energy you need for exercising. Water also helps your body regulate its temperature through sweating. Because vigorous exercise causes you to lose large amounts of water through sweating, it's important to drink water before, during, and after each workout session. Drink between eight and 16 ounces in the hour prior to working out. Replenish fluids by drinking four to eight ounces of every 15 minutes during your workout. During vigorous cardiovascular training, or if you're exercising in hot temperatures, increase your water consumption to replace water lost from sweating. Then, drink between eight and 16 ounces of water within 30 minutes of completing your exercise routine. Your muscles need water to recover from the stress of a workout. Drinking the right amounts after your workout will help reduce muscle soreness and help you feel less tired.

Hydrate right!

It's extremely important to stay fully hydrated before, during, and after your workout—just don't reach for a sports drink that is full of unwanted calories. While slews of TV commercials featuring famous pro athletes lead you to believe that sports drinks like Gatorade and Vitamin Water help you stay fit, these drinks actually contain up to 200 calories and 35 grams of carbs per bottle. The promise that these drinks will give you the energy and electrolytes you need to have a great workout is really just a marketing ploy. For instance, Gatorade was originally developed to help college football players avoid dehydration and cramping during a rigorous training program in the humid summer months. A normal person like you, who is exercising at a much more moderate level, has no need for the carbs and calories in a sports drink. Water is always your best option. If you like the flavoring in sports drinks, try a low or no-calorie version, like Powerade Zero or Gatorade's G2.

Don't overtrain

There is such a thing as too much exercise. Let's say you're preparing for a 5k race, and you start running several miles every day. You'll quickly notice that after a couple of weeks of training hard, your body begins to feel fatigued more quickly. You may find that you feel sore and even have trouble sleeping at night. These are symptoms of overtraining. In order to lose up to 10 pounds in 30 days, you will need to exercise daily; however, you shouldn't aim for a high-intensity cardio or weight-lifting session every day.

Did You Know?

Taking up long-distance running, cycling or swimming? Water is always a great choice for hydration and recovery, but what about the childhood favorite, chocolate milk? A study published in the *International Journal of Sport Nutrition and Exercise Metabolism* compared cyclists who consumed chocolate milk post-workout, and found they performed just as well, if not better, than those who drank other sports drinks during the next cycling session. Chocolate milk has high water content for hydrating the body, twice the carbs and protein for replenishing tired muscles, as well as calcium, which the other drinks lack.

It's not realistic or good for your body, which needs periods of rest and recovery. Build one or two "light days" into your weekly workout schedule, but make them count! Schedule the same amount of time for your workout as a normal day, just exercise at a lower intensity. Light days might include biking, walking, dynamic stretching (walking lunges or arm circles, for instance), and swimming. Keep your body in motion, but make sure you're giving hardworking muscle groups time to recover so you're full of energy and stamina for your next tough workout.

Work toward your target heart rate

If you're not working out within your target heart rate zone, you're not getting the maximum benefits. The "fat burning zone," which burns the most calories and body fat stores, is reached at about 60 to 70 percent of your maximum heart rate. To calculate your maximum heart rate, subtract your age from 226 (for women, 220 for men). Then, multiply that number by 0.6 (60 percent) or 0.7 (70 percent) to find the number of beats per minute that is your target heart rate.

To determine whether you're in that zone during your workout, either wear a heart rate monitor, or take your pulse for 10 seconds and multiply the number of beats by six. Adjust your intensity depending on whether you're above or below your target heart rate.

Exercise muscles in proper progression to maximize results

When you're working a variety of muscles during a strength training sequence, order is important. If your workout includes a variety of weight lifting exercises, begin with your larger muscle groups and move to the smaller ones. This allows for optimal performance of the most demanding exercises, as you want to have enough energy to complete your entire workout. It's better to do less and complete the entire circuit than to neglect a muscle group or do an uneven number of reps from one side of the body to the other.

Variety is the spice of life

Variety keeps you motivated in both your diet and your workouts. If you restrict yourself to eating only salads, for instance, you'll quickly lose interest and enthusiasm.

Variety also keeps your weight loss and calorie burning from plateauing. If you do the same exercises, at the same intensity, day after day, working out will get boring, and your body will stop burning fat and calories as quickly. You'll find your weight loss comes to a standstill. You need to plan for workouts that use different muscle groups at different intensities throughout the week. Because you're trying to torch unwanted pounds, you'll want to focus on cardio, but also complement it with strength training.

Chapter 9

Ultimate Fitness Tips

You're well on your way to a successful diet and fitness program and, by now, you're seeing the weight drop off, feeling healthier, and enjoying more energy than ever. To continue making progress, you need to keep your body from plateauing and your dedication from waning.

To round out your program, you need a few powerful secrets. In this chapter, learn how to exercise efficiently, stay inspired, and breeze through physical activity on a daily basis, without your workout feeling like "work."

Motivation, seeing results, and enjoyment are the keys to sticking with a fitness plan for 30 days, or any amount of time. This book has given you all the tools you need to lose up to 10 pounds and inches of belly fat faster than you ever thought possible—use this fitness chapter to rev up your workouts and get the very most from every minute of physical activity.

Make a music playlist to stay motivated

Music has been proven to help people work out longer and with more energy, as well as providing a distraction from fatigue. Dr. Costas Karageorghis, who has studied the effects of music on physical performance for 20 years, says that a good workout song should be between 120 and 140 beats-per-minute, which corresponds to the average person's heart rate while performing moderate exercise (up the tempo if you're working out harder). Most pop, rap, heavy metal, and rock songs fall into this tempo range. Even if it's not your favorite artist or a type of music that you'd listen to in your car, an upbeat song can help keep you going when your energy is low or you're nearing the end of a tough workout.

Invest in new workout clothes

When you feel confident and have the proper exercise clothes, you will be more motivated to exercise, and you'll work out longer, too. Invest in a few new pieces of workout clothing and you'll be inspired and excited to wear them! Choose shirts, shorts, pants, and sports bras in breathable, quick-drying fabrics that wick sweat away from the body. Exercise clothes should also stretch and move with you. Finally, be sure to get what you need for the specific activities you'll be engaging in, such as compression shorts for biking, form-fitting pants for yoga, and supportive undergarments for running.

Hydrate and replenish with coconut water

Coconut water is one of the purest natural liquids around, second only to real water. It's one of nature's best superfoods! Unlike sugary sports drinks, coconut water contains natural electrolytes for energy and hydration but with minimal calories (typically about 60 per bottle). Coconut water has no added sugar and, with more potassium than a banana and 15 times more than most sports drinks, it prevents cramping and promotes muscle recovery during and after a workout. It also has myriad weight-loss benefits, such as increasing metabolism and promoting healthy thyroid function.

You can buy individual servings of coconut water at most health food stores and at many gyms and fitness studios. Its natural properties and benefits to your health and exercise program make it a favorite of cyclists, runners, trainers, yogis, and more.

Use plyometrics to blast calories

Plyometrics are a great way to burn calories in a short amount of time, and are designed to produce fast, powerful movements. Plyometric exercises load the muscles and contract it in rapid sequence. When you do these exercises in succession they burn calories quickly. Plyometrics are efficient because they are strength-building exercises that require endurance and cardiovascular stamina.

You can try mixing jump rope, jumping jacks, squat jumps, box jumps, and other plyometric activities into your normal workouts. You can also refer to the *Sexy Abs Diet Pocket Guide* exercise plan chapter later in this book, which contains a complete, challenging plyometric and core workout.

Did You Know?
According to a *Men's Fitness* magazine survey of more than 5,000 readers, guys' favorite part of a woman's body is her butt (40 percent), beating out legs and even breasts! Guys preferred voluptuous bodies, like Kim Kardashian's, and athletic bodies, like Cameron Diaz's, over thin stick-figures. All the more motivation to define curves and build sexy muscles.

Get Netflix

No one is recommending you sit on your couch watching movies all night, but Netflix is actually a convenient, inexpensive way to work out at home! The wide selection of exercise and fitness DVDs includes dance, aerobics, yoga, Pilates, strength training, and more. Some DVDs are available for rental, delivered right to your mailbox, and can be kept as long as you like, and others can be watched instantly online, or on a gaming console like Wii or Xbox. Workout DVDs are perfect for the times when you need a quick, 30-minute blast, don't have time to drive to the gym, or want to try something new in the privacy of your living room. For example, maybe you're not sure if Hollywood trainer Jillian Michaels' *30-Day Shred* is right for you. Netflix gives you the option to try it before buying it. Just be sure to type in the name of the video you want into the Search bar—the "Browse" feature shows only a limited number of choices.

Find a fitness buddy

Losing weight and getting active are always easier with a partner, so invite a spouse or friend to join you in your weight-loss efforts, especially if he or she seems threatened by or uncomfortable with your weight loss. A workout buddy keeps you accountable, motivated on days when you don't feel like exercising, and provides you with company on hikes, bike rides, and rock climbing trips. Plus, if you're trying out a new form of exercise, such as surfing or kickboxing, having a partner can make it more fun and less scary. Make your workout buddy someone you see often, such as your neighbor, coworker, roommate, or spouse, and you'll be best able to hold each other accountable. And you'll have someone to celebrate with when you both drop 10 pounds!

Schedule a cardio session around a TV show or sporting event

Running or bicycling for an hour or more in a gym can get dull fast. One tip for getting through a longer cardio session is to plan it for a time when a favorite show, movie, or sporting event is on TV. Time will fly by when you're watching a Lakers game or a sitcom. Just be sure to do this when you have at least 45 minutes or more of cardio, so you can work at a steady pace and zone out a bit. You won't want the TV to distract you if you're trying to get through 30 minutes of interval training, for instance.

Get a boost from pre-workout caffeine

The caffeine in natural sources such as coffee, green tea, or in pill form, benefits your workouts because it acts as a thermogenic. Thermogenics speed up your body's functions, including breath and heart rate, encouraging the body to use calories more quickly. Don't overdo it when it comes to caffeine, of course. Listen to your body, and if you feel light-headed, dizzy, or faint, stop what you're doing immediately, rest for a few minutes, and abstain from caffeine in the future. Otherwise, unless you're exercising at high altitudes or suffer from high blood pressure or another heart condition, taking 100 to 200 mg (one cup of coffee has about 100 mg) of caffeine 45 minutes before a workout can help you burn fat stores, speed up your metabolism, and help you power through a workout.

Count your steps with a pedometer

Start wearing a pedometer daily to measure how many steps you're taking and how many calories you're burning. Pedometers clip to your belt or pocket—or any spot where they will be perpendicular to the ground. They come in a variety of styles and price points—for less than $20 you can get a sleek, simple device that counts steps and calculates calories burned. Deluxe models play music, have audio features, and allow you to upload your daily stats into your computer to track your progress and meet goals. Many new mp3 players come with built-in pedometers as well. You'll want to refer to consumer reports that test the efficiency and accuracy of different makes and models.

For $99, a Microsoft product called Fitbit accurately tracks your calories burned, steps taken, distance traveled, water intake, and even sleep quality. On your Fitbit profile, you enter the calories you ate for the day, and the data from your Fitbit device automatically calculates if you've met the distance and calorie goals you set for the day and week.

Blow off the gym!

Many people enjoy the routine schedule of going to the same location every day, but others find the gym stifling and somewhat limiting. Or you may feel lost among the confusing machines, bustling trainers, and intense gym rats. Be it burnout or pure intimidation, you may be looking for an alternative to the gym.

Naturally, getting outside in the fresh air is your best choice. If you live in a city where weather permits, add a fun activity to your weekly workout schedule—bike rides, hiking, surfing, horseback riding, rock climbing. Try something new to shake things up and stay motivated. Boot camps are also a great way to burn hundreds of calories in a short amount of time. Beach or park boot camps are popping up all over the country, as well as indoor sessions that combine strength training with cardio. Boot camps use interval training—bursts of activity with short rests in between exercises—to blast calories and fat. Another gym alternative is joining a private yoga or Pilates studio. You'll get focused, professional instructors and classes without the overwhelming nature of a gym atmosphere.

There are really hundreds of exercises, classes, and groups available. Check out the website MeetUp.com to find out what's going on in your area. From surfing moms to salsa dancing clubs, if you can imagine it, it's out there.

## Chapter 10

Activities & Calories Burned

All types of physical activity burn calories. You don't have to slave away at a gym—normal daily activities, such as chores and errands also burn calories.

This chapter highlights typical physical activities, from sports to household chores, that you can perform to burn calories. They range from light to moderate to vigorous, so incorporate something from each list every day, or combine activities.

Be aware that the exact number of calories you burn for each activity varies based on your weight. The following list is an approximation for someone who weighs 150 pounds. If you weigh more, you will burn slightly more calories; if you weigh less than 150 pounds, you will burn slightly fewer calories. If you require an exact count, there are many websites that can estimate calories burned based on your weight, intensity of the workout, and the length of time you exercised.

Light Activities: 150 or Less Cal/Hr.

Office work...140
Sitting 80
Standing.. 100

Moderate Activities: 150-350 Cal/Hr.

Bicycling (5 mph) 170
Dancing (social) 210
Gardening (moderate)...270
Golf (without cart)... 320
Horseback riding (sitting trot) 250
Light housework/cleaning, etc. 250
Surfing 300
Tennis (recreational doubles) 310
Walking (3 mph) 240

Vigorous Activities: 350 or More Cal/Hr.

Aerobics (step) 440
Basketball (leisure) 390
Bicycling (10 mph) 375
Cross country skiing (leisurely)............................. 460
Hiking 460
Ice skating (9 mph) 384
Rock climbing...740
Rollerblading 384
Running (8 mph)... 900
Shoveling snow 580
Soccer 580
Swimming (50 yards/min.)................................ 680
Yoga (power) 400

## Chapter 11

Exercise Plan

A sleeker, sexier you requires a fitness plan full of high-intensity, calorie-blasting exercises that work the whole body. The *Sexy Abs Diet Pocket Guide* exercise plan is designed to target multiple muscle groups, build core strength, and elevate the heart rate to burn body fat.

Six days out of each week you'll pair strength training with a cardio circuit. You'll need water, exercise shoes, and moveable, breathable workout clothes. Every day, you will do one of two core strength training sets, an upper body circuit, or a lower body circuit. For cardio, you can choose from a custom walking or running circuit, or pick your own activity. The seventh day of the week is to rest and recuperate.

Every strength training exercise comes with step-by-step instructions, as well as modifications to make the move easier or harder. You may want to challenge yourself more on some exercises, and modify other moves.

How to do the exercise plan

You will need about 60 minutes to complete this workout plan. Do each strength training exercise for 50 seconds, with as many reps as you can do in that time without sacrificing form. Take a 10-second rest. Keep your eye on a stopwatch or timer. Complete all six exercises in the strength training circuit, then repeat the full circuit for a second round, and again for a third. After you have completed three rounds of the strength training circuit, take a two-minute water break and move on to cardio.

Warming up and cooling down

Always begin and end your workouts with a five to 10-minute warm-up and cool-down. Walk or jog in place to loosen the muscles. Next, stretch to prepare your muscles for work and prevent injury. Important stretches include holding the heel close to the glute to stretch the quad muscle, reaching toward the toes to stretch hamstrings, and stretching your arms behind your head and across the chest to loosen shoulders, chest, and arms. The same routine after your workout will bring the heart rate down, help the body recover, and prevent soreness.

Work hard and push yourself, even if it's to do one more rep! You'll love the feeling of success and pride you'll get after a tough workout. The body, strength, and shape you've always wanted will be here in no time!

Core 1

Strength training is a very important part of losing weight. The following workout will slim, lengthen, and tone your core while replacing body fat with muscle, which burns three times as many calories as fat.

The exercises in this section work all parts of the core, including the abs, obliques, and lower back. You'll also work the arms, shoulders, and more. When coupled with a cardio program, these moves will help you get in shape quickly. Plus, they're fun and challenging!

Scorpion Plank

1. Start in plank position with hands under shoulders. Pull the right knee toward the left elbow and twist your torso to the left.

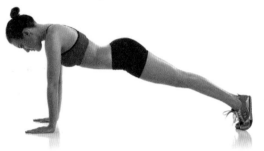

2. Return to starting position and switch sides, twisting the other side with the left leg. Keep your core engaged and don't let your hips sag.

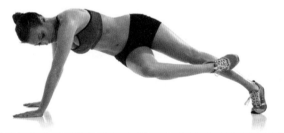

Make it easier: Bring the knee in to the chest and skip the twist.

Make it harder: Place your feet up on a stability ball to force the core to work even harder.

Crunch on a Stability Ball

1. Start with your shoulders, lower back, and hips on a stability ball. Interlace your fingers behind your head, and pull your belly button in toward your spine.

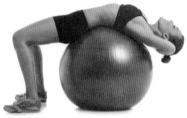

2. Raise your head and shoulders in a crunch, pausing at the top, and returning slowly to a start position.

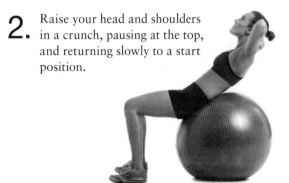

Make it easier: Crunch on the ground without the stability ball.

Make it harder: Hold a dumbbell in both hands as you crunch.

Hip Crossover with Stability Ball

1. Rest your feet on a stability ball with knees bent, so the ball is resting against the back of the thighs. Arms should be straight out to the sides.

2. Squeezing the ball against the backs of the thighs and engaging the core, drop the ball to the right side as low as you can without lifting your shoulders off the floor.

3. Reverse the movement all the way to the left side, without pausing in the middle, to complete one rep. Then return to center and repeat.

Make it easier: Don't lower as close to the ground.

Make it harder: Move slowly and with control.

Side Plank with Push-up

1. Start in plank position.

2. Flip to one side; straighten your bottom arm directly under your shoulder, legs straight, and feet stacked. Place your free hand on your hip or stretch it up. Keep your back straight and do not allow your hips to sag. Work on tightening your abs and lifting your side away from the ground.

3. Flip back to plank and complete a push-up for one rep on that side. Repeat, switching sides.

Make it easier: Place one knee on the ground. Skip the push-up.

Make it harder: Lift the top leg up six inches.

Reverse Crunch

1. Lie on your back with your arms by your sides. Keep your palms pressed into the floor, and bend your knees at about a 90-degree angle.

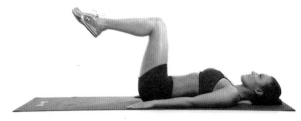

2. Lift your pelvis, using the lower abs, and hollow out the belly. Your knees should come slightly in toward your head. Pause at the top of the crunch, then lower the legs just above the floor, for one rep.

Make it easier: Keep the range of motion smaller. Don't lift hips as high or lower legs as low to the ground.

Make it harder: Perform with straight legs. Lower legs toward the ground slowly and with control.

Russian Twist with Dumbbell

1. Sit upright with your legs bent and feet on the floor. Hold arms out in front of you and hold a dumbbell with both hands. Lean slightly back so your upper body forms a 45-degree angle with the floor.

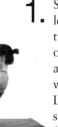

2. Rotate your arms and the dumbbell as far to one side as you can, reaching down while you squeeze your abs and obliques.

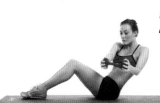

3. Return to center and twist to the other side. Rotate from your core, not your hips.

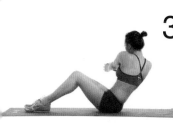

Make it easier: Don't use a dumbbell.

Make it harder: Lift your feet off the floor and don't let them touch at any time.

Notes:

_____

_____

_____

_____

_____

_____

_____

_____

_____

_____

_____

_____

_____

_____

_____

_____

_____

_____

_____

Core 2

This second set of core exercises will whip your middle into shape in just 30 days. You'll feel leaner and stronger, especially when you combine these moves with a cardio program.

Don't forget to challenge yourself as much as possible, and modify as necessary to push yourself or account for injuries or sore muscles.

Bird Dog

1. Start in a table position, with your hands and knees on the floor, shoulder-width apart. Keep your core engaged so the hips don't sag and the back doesn't arch.

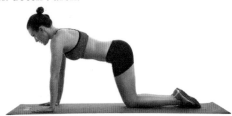

2. Raise your right arm out in front and your left leg back simultaneously, keeping them in line with your torso. Hold for a second, then return to the starting position. Repeat with the opposite arm and leg.

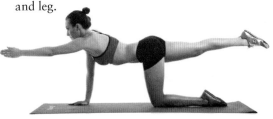

Make it easier: Raise your arm or leg separately. Hold for a second, then return to starting position.

Make it harder: While your arm and leg are raised as high as you can, add three pulse ups before returning to start position.

Jackknife and Push-up on Stability Ball

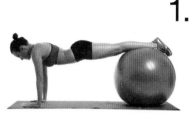

1. Begin in a plank position with your hands under your shoulders and the tops of the feet and shins elevated on a stability ball.

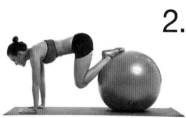

2. Without rounding the lower back, bend your knees and use your core muscles to pull the ball in to the body.

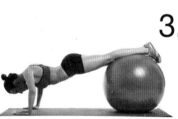

3. Push the ball back out to plank, then lower into a push-up to complete a rep.

Make it easier: Skip the push-up.

Make it harder: Instead of bending your knees, keep the legs straight and lift your hips up so you end up in a pike position.

Side Bend with Dumbbell

1. Stand straight with your feet shoulder-width apart, holding a dumbbell in each hand, palms facing your sides.

2. Keeping your back straight and bending only at the waist, bend to one side as far as you can, feeling your oblique muscles engage on both sides. Then return to the starting position and repeat. Repeat on the same side, switching sides at the 25-second mark.

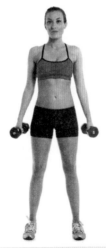 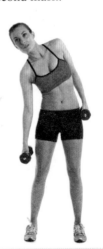

Make it easier: Use a lighter weight or don't use a dumbbell.

Make it harder: Use a heavier weight.

X Sit-ups

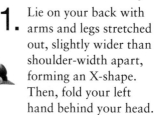

1. Lie on your back with arms and legs stretched out, slightly wider than shoulder-width apart, forming an X-shape. Then, fold your left hand behind your head.

2. Sit straight up, pointing your right hand up above the head, as if you are reaching for the ceiling.

3. Next, crunch forward, reaching the right hand across the body to touch the left toe. Reverse the movement and lie back down, for one rep. Switch arms and repeat on the opposite side.

Make it easier: Point both hands out in front of you and crunch with this modified arm position.

Make it harder: Sit cross-legged to force the core to work harder. Engage the core and don't let your lower back hunch over.

Bicycles

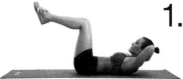

1. Lie on your back with your knees bent at a 90-degree angle.

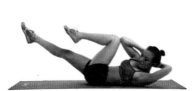

2. Lace your fingers behind your head. Lift your head and shoulders, exhale, and twist to one side, bringing your knee in to touch your opposite elbow, while straightening the other leg. Return to center and inhale.

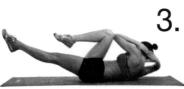

3. Exhale and twist to the opposite side.

Make it easier: Keep feet on the ground and slide heels along the floor using a towel.

Make it harder: Perform bicycles as fast as you can, being sure to rotate from the core.

Rollout on a Stability Ball

1. Kneel in front of a stability ball. Interlace your fingers tightly and place your fist on the top of the ball.

2. Keeping your core engaged, slowly roll the ball out and away from you, straightening your arms as much as you can without sagging your hips or collapsing through the lower back. Use your abs to pull you back to the starting position.

Make it easier: Keep the ball closer to the body.

Make it harder: Push the ball out further and keep the ball under your wrists.

Upper Body

These upper body exercises work different parts of your chest, back, shoulders, as well as upper and lower arms.

Challenge yourself, but don't sacrifice form. It's better to do fewer high-quality reps than more reps with bad form.

Judo Push-ups

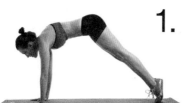

1. Put your hands and feet flat on the ground, with your hips lifted so your body forms an inverted V shape.

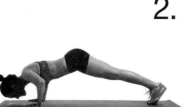

2. Keeping your hips up, bend your arms out to the side, and lower your upper body until your chin is near the floor.

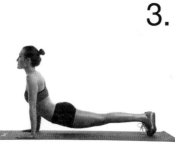

3. Lower your hips toward the floor while you lift your upper body simultaneously. Then slide back into the original position, reversing the way you went in, for one rep.

Make it easier: Put your knees on the ground as your lower your hips to the floor.

Make it harder: Lift one leg.

Chest Fly on Stability Ball

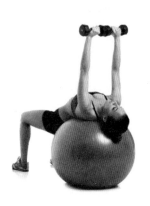

1. Lie in a table position with your shoulders and upper back on a stability ball and feet on the floor, hip-width apart. Hold a dumbbell in each hand, above your chest, palms facing out. Keep your core engaged and your hips lifted.

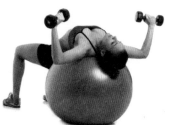

2. With slightly bent elbows, lower your arms down and back. Don't let arms go below chest-height. Press arms back up, and touch to complete one rep.

Make it easier: Use lighter weights.

Make it harder: Use heavier weights, but don't sacrifice form.

Bent Row

1. Stand with feet shoulder-width apart, holding a dumbbell in each hand, palms facing your thighs. Hinge forward at the hips, so your torso is parallel or almost parallel to the floor.

2. Bend at the elbows, pulling arms straight back until weights are at chest-height. Squeeze the shoulder blades at the top of the row; then lower your arms for one rep.

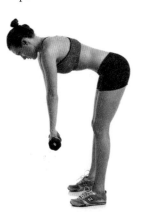
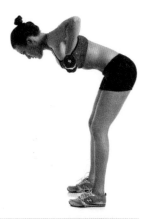

Make it easier: Use a lighter weight.

Make it harder: Extend one leg behind you into an arabesque as you hinge forward, forming a T with your body. You will use your abs and glutes to maintain balance.

Seated Tricep Extensions

1. Sit on a stability ball, holding a dumbbell at one end in both hands, with hands overlapping one another. Then extend the arms overhead with arms by the ears.

2. Lower the dumbbell behind your head until arms reach about a 90-degree angle. Then press the arms back up to straight. Keep the core engaged to avoid arching your back.

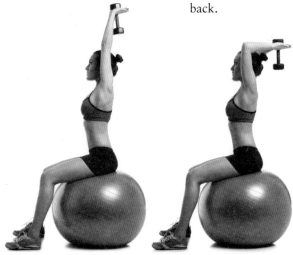

Make it easier: **Use a lighter weight.**

Make it harder: **Use a heavier weight.**

Dumbbell Swing

1. Hold a dumbbell with an overhand grip (palm facing toward the body) between your legs; bend your knees and squat down.

2. Thrusting through your glutes and hips, and squeezing the shoulders, stand up and swing the dumbbell up until it is chest-high.

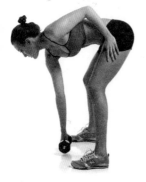

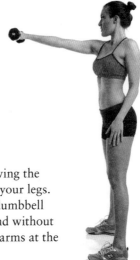

3. Squat back down and swing the dumbbell back between your legs. Continue swinging the dumbbell back and forth fluidly and without sacrificing form. Switch arms at the 25-second mark.

Make it easier: **Hold the dumbbell with two hands.**

Make it harder: **Use a heavier weight, but don't sacrifice form.**

Close Chest Press on Ball

1. Lie back so your feet are on the floor, about hip-width apart, and your upper back is resting on a stability ball, forming a table position. Hold a set of dumbbell directly over your chest, palms facing each other, with the dumbbells touching.

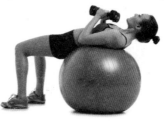

2. Lower the set of dumbbells to the center of your chest, then press them back up to the starting position for one rep. If this exercise is too difficult, you can alternate arms one at a time.

Make it easier: Spread your feet wide to help stabilize your body.

Make it harder: Keep your feet close together to make your stabilizer muscles work harder.

Windmill with Dumbbell

1. Stand with feet just wider than shoulders, toes turned out slightly. Hold dumbbell in left hand with arms extended out to the side at shoulder height. Slowly bend torso to the right, bringing right arm toward the floor and left arm toward sky.

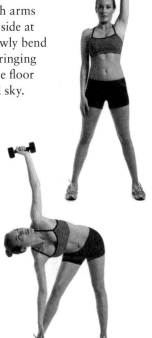

2. Keep your eyes on the weight in your extended arm; then reverse the movement to get back upright. Switch sides halfway through.

Make it easier: Use a lighter weight or no weight.

Make it harder: Use a heavier but manageable weight.

Lower Body

Equipment:
Stability ball
Dumbbells

This series of lunges, raises, and plyometric moves will whip your thighs, hamstrings, glutes, and calves into shape in no time! You'll feel stronger and more explosive throughout the entire lower body.

A lower body circuit combined with cardio work can be a lot on the legs, so be sure to walk for a few minutes or jog in place to warm up the body completely. And remember, concentrate on using proper form to make the most of these moves.

Side Lunge With Chop

1. Stand with legs shoulder-width apart and toes slightly turned out, holding a dumbbell on both ends at chest-height.

2. Lunge out to the left side and bring the dumbbell across the front of the body and down toward the outer edge of the foot.

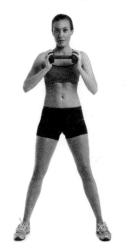

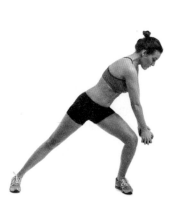

3. Press back up through the foot and thigh to return to a standing position. Repeat until the 25-second mark where you will switch sides.

Make it easier: **Use a lighter dumbbell.**

Make it harder: **Use a heavier dumbbell.**

Lunges with a Twist

1. Start standing, then step forward into a lunge, making sure your knee doesn't go past your toes.

2. When you reach the lowest point of your lunge, twist your torso to the side of the leg that is up, squeezing the core. Stand up from the lunge and repeat on the other leg.

Make it easier: Don't sink as low in your lunge.

Make it harder: Lunge holding a dumbbell in front of your chest for extra difficulty.

Sumo Squats with Dumbbell

1. Stand with feet about twice as wide as your shoulders, toes turned out slightly, holding a dumbbell in both hands at waist height.

2. Squat as low as you can, keeping a natural arch in the lower back, as if you are going to touch the weight to the ground between your feet.

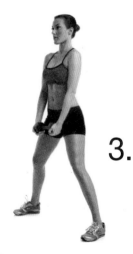

3. Come back up to the starting position and repeat. Keep the core engaged, focus the weight into your heels, and squeeze your glutes as you rise, pushing through the toes to work the calves as well.

Make it easier: Skip the weight.

Make it harder: As you come up to standing position, lift the weight over your head until your arms are straight, for one complete rep.

Twisting Arabesque

1. In your right hand, hold a light dumbbell on one end. Stand with your arms at your sides. Place your right toe on the floor about a foot behind you.

2. Bend forward from the hips. Keeping your right leg straight, raise it off the floor until your body forms a T, and your arms hang straight down from your shoulders. Your left knee can have a slight bend for stability.

3. As you bend forward, twist from the core and reach across the body so the dumbbell in your right hand comes down toward your left foot. Return to the starting position. Switch legs and hold the dumbbell in the other hand at the 25-second mark.

Make it easier: Do not use a dumbbell.

Make it harder: Reach down until you touch the weight to your foot.

Clamshell with Dumbbell

1. Lie on your side with your knees slightly bent and legs and heels together. Rest your head against the crook of your elbow. Keep your top arm against your hip and leg, holding a dumbbell comfortably against the hip area to create resistance and added difficulty.

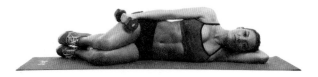

2. Keeping your feet and heels together, raise your top knee as high as you can, mimicking the shape of a clamshell. Pause at the top of the movement, then lower to start position. Switch sides at the 25-second mark.

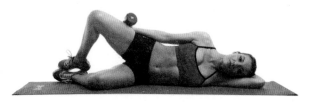

Make it easier: **Do not use a dumbbell.**

Make it harder: **Use a heavier weight.**

Crossover Lunge & Press

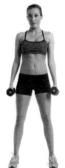

1. Stand with your feet hip-width apart. Hold two dumbbells with your arms straight down, palms facing toward your sides.

2. Keeping your back upright and hips and shoulders square, take a big step back with your right leg, crossing it behind your left. Bend your knees and lower your hips until your left thigh is nearly parallel to the floor.

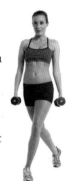

3. At the bottom of the lunge, press the dumbbells up overhead to touch end to end, palms facing outward. Lower the dumbbells and step up from the lunge to return to the starting position.

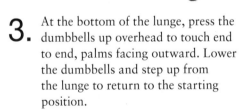

Make it easier: Use a lighter weight or skip the overhead press.

Make it harder: Use a heavier weight or sink deeper in the crossover lunge, as long as the knee doesn't come past the foot.

Cardio Plan

Equipment:
None

Combining strength training with cardiovascular exercise is the best way to lose weight quickly, safely, and easily. After performing the core, upper, or lower body exercises prescribed for the day, choose a cardio activity. The cardio portion of this plan includes one running and one walking interval for blasting calories in a short amount of time; choose from one of those custom programs, or pick your own cardio activity of 30 minutes or more.

Whatever you choose, from walking to hiking to kickboxing to surfing, be sure the activity is vigorous enough to get your heart rate up. When you reach your target heart rate, which is 60 to 70 percent of your maximum heart rate, you are in the zone where your body burns the most calories and body fat stores.

Cardio Pyramid

This cardio workout will take 30 minutes. You will combine shorts bursts of jogging, running, and sprinting with periods of active recovery. You can adjust speeds as needed, but try to challenge yourself. Active recovery can be either a gentle jog or walk. Sprinting should be running almost as fast as you can. For an extra challenge, you can do this workout where there are uphill sections.

TIME	ACTIVITY	RECOVER
5 min.	walk or jog	0
1 min.	run	1
30 sec.	sprint	30 sec.
15 sec.	sprint	15 sec.
1 min.	run	1
1 min.	sprint	1
3.5 min.	jog or run	3.5
1 min.	sprint	1
1 min.	run	1
15 sec.	sprint	15 sec.
30 sec.	sprint	30 sec.
1 min.	run	1
5 min.	walk or jog	0

Walking Hills Workout

Walking is low-impact but still packs a calorie-burning punch, especially when walking at various speeds. A slow walk is for warming up and periods of active recovery. A moderate walk should get your heart rate up and have you moving briskly. A fast walk should mean you are working your hardest, raising your heart rate, and feeling a burn in the legs and glutes. Be sure to pump your arms and keep your core tight and back straight. Here is a 30-minute walking workout you can do anywhere.

MINUTES	ACTIVITY
5	warm up
2	moderate walk
2	fast walk
1	slow walk
1	fast walk
4	moderate walk
2	slow walk
2	fast walk
3	moderate walk
3	fast walk
5	cool down

Group Class, Activity, or Sport
of Your Choice

You may also choose the physical activity you want to engage in as your cardio for the day. Be sure to challenge yourself and do an activity, class, or sport that lasts 30 to 60 minutes and gets your heart rate up, such as:

MINUTES	ACTIVITY
30-60	Cardio kickboxing class
30-60	Swimming
30-60	Challenging hike
30-60	Vigorous bike ride
30-60	Surfing
30-60	Tennis
30-60	Yoga flow class
30-60	Aerobics class
30-60	Spinning
30-60	Running/climbing stairs

## Chapter 12

Meal Plan

The *Sexy Abs Diet Pocket Guide* meal plan has been custom-created by our registered dietician and nutrition specialist, Lindsey Toth, to provide healthy breakfasts, lunches, and dinners. Each meal contains about 400 calories, with a balance of carbohydrates, healthy fats, protein, and fiber to help you slim down, de-bloat, increase energy, and feel satiated. With the nutritional information for each meal broken down, recording your daily caloric intake in your journal is easy. Best of all, every meal is simple to make, includes ingredients anyone can find, and tastes delicious.

Toth, MS, RD, is a nationally recognized registered dietician and nutritionist for PepsiCo's Global Nutrition Communications Team. She holds degrees from Michigan State University and Tufts University in clinical nutrition and nutrition communications. Her expertise has been tapped for *Redbook*, *Nutrition Today*, *The Dr. Oz Show*, and more.

Apple Strudel Oatmeal

Prep Time: 7 minutes, **Total Time:** 10 minutes

Did your mom ever tell you no dessert for breakfast? Well we're flipping that rule on its head. Warm, sweet, and ever so delicious, this oatmeal is the perfect start to your day.

Ingredients:

- ½ cup dried, old-fashioned oats
- 1 cup fat-free milk
- ½ apple, cored, and diced
- ½ tsp cinnamon
- ½ tsp brown sugar
- 2 tbsps of crushed & roasted unsalted pecans

Directions:

1. Portion dried oatmeal into a bowl and mix in milk, cinnamon, and brown sugar.

2. Stir in diced apple and microwave on high for 3 minutes, stirring occasionally.

3. Mix in crushed pecans and enjoy!

Did You Know?

There are more than 7,500 varieties of apples grown in the world, and about 2,500 varieties grown in the United States. Each variety has its own unique flavor (Fuji are sweet, Braeburn are tart, etc.), so test out different kinds in your oatmeal to find the taste that's right for you!

Nutrition Information:

371 calories
56 g carbohydrates
8 g fiber
15 g protein
11 g fat
1 g saturated fat

Huevos Rancheros

Prep Time: 6 minutes, **Total Time:** 20 minutes

This is a classic Mexican breakfast dish, with a low calorie twist. Try this recipe on a weekend morning, or a morning when you have enough time to get your oven going.

Directions:

1. Preheat oven to 400°F.

2. Combine beans, lime juice, cumin, and olive oil in a small bowl.

3. Spray both sides of tortilla with olive oil cooking spray and bake in oven until crisp, about 10 minutes.

4. Spray frying pan lightly with olive oil cooking spray and add in eggs. Cook until whites are set, about 3 minutes.

5. Plate egg on top of tortilla, and top with beans, avocado, salsa, and cilantro.

Ingredients:

- 2 eggs
- 1 La Tortilla Factory 100% Whole Wheat 50 Calorie Tortilla
- ⅛ cup canned black beans, rinsed to remove excess sodium
- ½ tsp lime juice
- ¾ tsp olive oil
- ⅛ tsp ground cumin
- ¼ cup salsa
- ¼ of 1 avocado, peeled, pitted, and sliced
- Olive oil cooking spray
- 1 tsp cilantro

Nutrition Information:
313 calories,
25 g carbohydrates,
9 g fiber, 17 g protein,
18 g fat, 4 g saturated fat

BREAKFAST

South of the Border Breakfast Sandwich

Prep Time: 7 minutes, **Total Time:** 10 minutes

This breakfast gem has all the magical zing of a breakfast burrito without the supersized portion and crazy calories. And, the lean turkey will keep you focused and satisfied until lunch.

Ingredients:

- 1 whole wheat English muffin
- 2 oz 98% fat-free deli turkey (usually 3-4 slices or 56 grams)
- 3 egg whites (or the equivalent in carton egg substitutes)
- 1 tbsp of shredded, low-fat mozzarella cheese
- ¼ cup fresh baby spinach leaves (or ⅛ cup thawed frozen spinach)
- 1 tbsp salsa
- Olive oil cooking spray

Directions:

1. Cut English muffin in half and place in toaster until toasted.

2. While muffin is toasting, pour egg whites in a small bowl, whisking in mozzarella with a fork. Add spinach and stir completely.

3. Spray a coffee mug with cooking spray and pour egg mixture into mug.

4. Microwave egg mixture on high for 1:30 to 2 minutes, checking occasionally until done (eggs should form a slightly domed patty shape when done).

5. Remove egg cup from microwave and place egg patty on one side of toasted English muffin. Place turkey slices on other side and top with salsa. Put halves together and enjoy!

Nutrition Information:
371 calories, 56 g carbohydrates, 8 g fiber, 15 g protein, 11 g fat, 1 g saturated fat

Tomato Muffin Breakfast Pizza

Prep Time: 3 minutes, **Total Time:** 8 minutes

This savory breakfast recipe is good mix-up to the traditional cereal you may be having, and is chock-full of fiber and flavor.

Directions:

1. Cut English muffin in half.

2. Spread with ricotta cheese, top with tomato halves, and sprinkle with salt and pepper to taste.

3. Toast in toaster or conventional oven for 4-5 minutes, or until crispy.

Ingredients:

- 1 whole wheat English muffin
- 6 cherry tomatoes, cut in half
- 4 tbsps fat-free ricotta cheese
- ½ tsp dried basil
- Salt and pepper to taste

Did You Know?

Why is breakfast the most important meal of the day? The word breakfast literally means "breaking the fast of the night," as it's the first meal taken after a night's sleep. This meal is needed to restock our body's energy stores, which have been depleted during the night, so we have energy for the day ahead.

Nutrition Information:

199 calories
35 g carbohydrates
7 g fiber
13 g protein
1 g fat
0 g saturated fat

Zesty Pepper Packed Breakfast Roll-Up

Prep Time: 5 minutes, **Total Time:** 8 minutes

Packed with colorful peppers, this breakfast wrap is full of fiber, vitamin A, and B vitamins. It's also a snap to put together, and best of all, it's great if you're on-the-go!

Ingredients:

- 1 La Tortilla Factory 100% Whole Wheat 100 Calorie Tortilla
- ¾ cup carton egg substitutes, like Egg Beaters (or 3 egg whites)
- 1 slice fat-free, white American cheese
- 1 cup frozen bell pepper, stir fry mix, reheated in microwave
- ¼ tsp red pepper
- 2 tbsps salsa
- Olive oil cooking spray

Directions:

1. Spray a coffee mug or small bowl with cooking spray, and pour egg whites into it.

2. Microwave eggs on high for 1:30 to 2 minutes, stirring occasionaly until done to form a scramble.

3. Remove egg scramble from microwave and spread eggs onto one side of open tortilla, sprinkling with red pepper. Top with bell pepper mix, cheese, and salsa.

4. Roll into burrito form and microwave on high for another 15-20 seconds to melt cheese, and serve.

Nutrition Information:
258 calories
37 g carbohydrates
10 g fiber
29 g protein
2 g fat
0 g saturated fat

Mean Green Breakfast Smoothie

Prep Time: 2 minutes, **Total Time:** 7 minutes

The color of this smoothie may be a bit off-putting, but the nutritional benefits aren't. This smoothie is chock-full of cancer-fighting phytochemicals and anthocyanins.

Directions:

1. Combine milk, yogurt, berries, sweet potato, and spinach in a blender.

2. Blend until smooth.

3. Pour into glass and enjoy.

Ingredients:

- 1 cup fat-free milk
- 1 6-oz container of nonfat vanilla Greek yogurt
- ½ cup mixed, frozen berries
- ¼ raw sweet potato
- 1 cup chopped, frozen spinach

Did You Know?

Fresh spinach slowly loses its nutritional value after harvested. While fresh, its leaves are crisp and vibrant, but as it deteriorates, the leaves turn limp. Freeze spinach while fresh to preserve its high nutrient profile.

Nutrition Information:

319 calories
49 g carbohydrates
7 g fiber
31 g protein
1 g fat
0 g saturated fat

Fresh Berry Crêpes

Prep Time: 5 minutes, **Total Time:** 12 minutes

Think you have to head to France for crêpes? Think again! This meal is a fun and exotic way to incorporate fruit into your morning routine, and is a good source of B vitamins and fiber.

Ingredients:

- ¼ cup whole wheat flour
- 1 egg white (or ¼ cup egg substitute, like Egg Beaters)
- ¼ cup fat-free milk
- 1 ½ tsps cinnamon applesauce
- Dash of salt
- ½ tsp vanilla extract
- ½ cup mixed frozen berries, thawed
- Pinch of powdered sugar
- Cooking spray

Nutrition Information:
204 calories
37 g carbohydrates
8 g fiber
13 g protein
1 g fat
0 g saturated fat

Directions:

1. In a small bowl, whisk together flour, egg, milk, applesauce, salt, and vanilla until smooth.

2. Heat frying pan on medium heat. Spray lightly with cooking spray to coat when heated.

3. Pour ½ of batter into skillet.

4. Tilt pan in circular motion to spread batter to edges, and cook until bottom is light brown, about 2 minutes.

5. Flip crêpe and fill with thawed mixed berries. Cook for another 2 minutes.

6. Fold crêpe in half and transfer to a plate.

7. Repeat with other half of batter for a second crêpe.

8. Dust crêpes lightly with powdered sugar and serve.

Cinnamon Pumpkin Swirl Yogurt Parfait

Prep Time: 0 minutes, **Total Time:** 3 minutes

This parfait brings the spirit of fall straight into your kitchen, with antioxidant rich spices like cinnamon and nutmeg, as well as nutrient packed pumpkin and yogurt.

Directions:

1. Scoop yogurt into a small bowl.

2. Stir in cinnamon, honey, vanilla, and pumpkin.

3. Top with almonds and oats, sprinkle with nutmeg, and enjoy!

Ingredients:

- 6 oz non-fat plain Greek yogurt (¾ cup)
- ¼ tsp ground cinnamon
- 1 ½ tsps honey
- ¼ tsp vanilla
- 1 tbsp canned raw pumpkin
- 1 tbsp old fashioned oats
- 1 tbsp sliced almonds
- Dash of nutmeg

Did You Know?

Research has shown that cinnamon has the highest antioxidant level of any of the spices, and even higher than many foods. There are as many antioxidants in 1 teaspoon of cinnamon as there are in an entire cup of pomegranate juice and as many as there are in ½ cup of blueberries!

Nutrition Information:

322 calories
35 g carbohydrates
5 g fiber
25 g protein
11 g fat
1 g saturated fat

Avocado Breakfast Toast

Prep Time: 10 minutes, **Total Time:** 15 minutes

Avocados are loaded with heart-healthy unsaturated fat, vitamins C, K, folate, and B6, and potassium. Why not get your fix with this delicious breakfast toast?

Ingredients:

- 2 slices of whole wheat bread, toasted
- 2 tbsps Dijon honey mustard
- ½ avocado, peeled and sliced
- ½ tomato, thinly sliced
- 1 tablespoon of dried basil
- Salt and pepper to taste

Directions:

1. Spread 1 tablespoon of the Dijon honey mustard on each piece of toast.

2. Add the avocado and the tomato slices evenly to each slice of toast.

3. Sprinkle both slices with basil and the salt and pepper to taste.

4. Eat with caution–this can get messy but it's definitely worth it!!

Did You Know?

The avocado is actually a fruit. Avocados provide nearly 20 essential nutrients to our bodies, including fiber, potassium, folic acid, vitamin E, and B vitamins, and also help our bodies absorb fat-soluble nutrients like alpha and beta-carotene.

Nutrition Information:

351 calories
45 g carbohydrates
12 g fiber
11 g protein
16 g fat
2 g saturated fat

Corn and Cheese Frittata

Prep Time: 10 minutes, Total Time: 18 minutes

This frittata is a delicious mixture of eggs and veggies, low in saturated fat, and high in B vitamins and vitamin A. Add in 34 grams of protein, and you're set to rock that morning meeting.

Directions:

1. Heat broiler-proof skillet over medium heat. Stir in olive oil, corn, zucchini, green onions, and tomatoes. Sauté for 3-5 minutes until vegetables are tender.

2. In a small bowl, mix together eggs and basil.

3. Pour egg mixture over vegetables in pan. As mixture sets, lift cooked portions so uncooked eggs flow underneath. Continue cooking until almost set. Sprinkle with cheese.

4. Place skillet in oven under broiler for 1-2 minutes or until top is set and cheese is melted.

Ingredients:

- 1 cup egg substitutes, like Egg Beaters
- 1 tsp olive oil
- ⅓ cup whole corn kernels
- ⅓ cup chopped zucchini
- ⅛ cup sliced green onions
- ⅓ cup diced tomatoes
- ⅛ cup fat-free cheddar cheese
- Olive oil cooking spray

Nutrition Information:
284 calories
27 g carbohydrates
4 g fiber
34 g protein
6 g fat
1 g saturated fat

Banana Split Smoothie

Prep Time: 2 minutes, Total Time: 7 minutes

This may seem reminiscent of a banana split, but the protein it's packing is definitely not. With 17 grams to fill you up, it keeps you satisfied until lunch time.

Ingredients:

- 1 cup fat-free milk
- ½ cup mixed, frozen strawberries
- 1 banana
- 2 tbsps peanut butter
- 2 tbsps no sugar added Nesquik

Directions:

1. Combine milk, berries, banana, peanut butter, and Nesquik powder in a blender.

2. Blend until smooth.

3. Pour into glass and enjoy.

Did You Know?

The browner the banana is, the sweeter it tastes. If some of your bananas are going brown, throw them in the freezer instead of the trash, and save them for smoothies. When you're ready to make your smoothie, remove the banana from the freezer, microwave it for 15-20 seconds, rip off the tip, and just squeeze the thawed banana into your blender.

Nutrition Information:

375 calories
44 g carbohydrates
6 g fiber
17 g protein
17 g fat
4 g saturated fat

Fruit & Yogurt Roll-Up

Prep Time: 2 minutes, Total Time: 8 minutes

Not feeling like a savory, egg and cheese breakfast burrito? This fruit and yogurt burrito is the perfect solution: sweet, crunchy, and packed with protein.

Directions:

1. Spread cream cheese on tortilla. Top with Greek yogurt, oats, and nuts.

2. Microwave berries to thaw if still frozen and add to tortilla.

3. Roll tightly to prevent yogurt spillage, and enjoy.

Ingredients:

- 1 La Tortilla Factory 100% Whole Wheat 100 Calorie Tortilla
- ½ oz fat-free cream cheese
- 3 oz fat-free vanilla Greek yogurt
- 1 tbsp dried, old-fashioned oats
- 1 tbsp crushed walnuts
- 1 cup of frozen mixed berries, thawed

Did You Know?

Greek yogurt can contain up to four times the amount of protein as regular yogurt, and can be easier on the stomach for those with lactose-intolerance, as it has less lactose. Stick with the non-fat variety for a rich and creamy yogurt that's sure to satisfy both your taste buds and your waistline.

Nutrition Information:
363 calories
57 g carbohydrates
17 g fiber
26 g protein
7 g fat
1 g saturated fat

Cranberry Peanut Butter English Muffin

Prep Time: 0 minutes, **Total Time:** 6 minutes

Cut the traditional butter out of your muffin routine and replace it with protein-packed peanut butter. And the whole wheat muffin delivers a healthy dose of fiber.

Ingredients:

- 1 whole wheat English muffin
- 2 tbsps unsalted peanut butter
- 2 tbsps dried cranberries

Directions:

1. Cut English muffin in half and spread each side with 1 tbsp of peanut butter.

2. Top each half with 1 tbsp of dried cranberries.

3. Toast in toaster or traditional oven until crispy and serve.

Did You Know?

Looking to break away from your traditional peanut butter? Try mixing it up this morning with a different kind of nut butter, like almond or walnut butter. Both nut butters are as high in protein as peanut butter, and lower in saturated fat.

Nutrition Information:

370 calories
47 g carbohydrates
7 g fiber
13 g protein
17 g fat
3 g saturated fat

Tropical Sunrise Oatmeal

Prep Time: 3 minutes, **Total Time:** 6 minutes

Is the cold weather giving you the vacation blues? Or maybe you want to celebrate summertime with an equally festive breakfast. Either way, this breakfast bowl is the perfect solution.

Directions:

1. Portion dried oatmeal into a bowl and mix in milk, vanilla extract, and pineapple.

2. Microwave on high for 3 minutes, stirring occasionally.

3. Mix in shredded coconut and enjoy!

Ingredients:

- ½ cup dried, old-fashioned oats
- 1 cup fat-free milk
- ½ cup canned pineapple, drained
- ¼ tsp vanilla extract
- 2 tbsps dried, sweetened, shredded coconut

Did You Know?

Some canned fruit, like canned pineapple, comes packed in syrup. This can significantly increase the calories you're consuming. When buying canned fruit, look for fruit that is canned in 100% juice for extra calorie savings. Want a flavor spin? Try using canned peaches, pears, or mandarin oranges instead of pineapple.

Nutrition Information:

337 calories
56 g carbohydrates
6 g fiber
14 g protein
7 g fat
4 g saturated fat

Cereal Sundae

Prep Time: 0 minutes, **Total Time:** 3 minutes

A sundae for breakfast? In this case, absolutely! This breakfast sundae is full of fiber, calcium, and protein, perfect for your early morning wake-up call.

Ingredients:

- 6 oz non-fat vanilla Greek yogurt (¾ cup)
- ½ cup bran flake cereal, like Raisin Bran
- 1 tbsp sliced almonds
- 1 tbsp dried cranberries

Directions:

1. Scoop yogurt into a small bowl.

2. Stir in bran cereal, almonds, and cranberries.

3. Serve and enjoy.

Did You Know?

Almonds are one of the best food sources of vitamin E, and are a high source of calcium, magnesium, potassium, as well as a natural source of protein and fiber. A 1-ounce serving has 13 grams of good unsaturated fats, helping you maintain heart health.

Nutrition Information:

310 calories
43 g carbohydrates
5 g fiber
21 g protein
8 g fat
1 g saturated fat

Fresh Peach & Chicken Spinach Salad

Prep Time: 10 minutes, **Total Time:** 15 minutes

Not only is it tasty, but this fresh and flavorful dish is also rich in vitamins A, C, and K, and low in calories to help you reach those weight-loss goals.

Directions:

1. Plate spinach leaves and top with peach cubes, chicken, and cucumber.

2. In a small bowl or dressing container, thoroughly mix together vinegar, lemon juice, sugar, mint, and salt.

3. Top chicken salad mixture with dressing, toss to coat, and serve.

Ingredients:

- 3 oz cooked, cubed chicken breast (about ½ cup)
- 1 small peach, pitted and cubed
- ¼ of one medium cucumber, cubed
- 1 cup fresh baby spinach leaves

Vinaigrette:

- 1 tbsp white wine vinegar
- ¾ tsp lemon juice
- 1 tbsp sugar
- 1 tbsp fresh mint
- ⅛ tsp salt
- ⅛ tsp pepper

Nutrition Information:

368 calories
45 g carbohydrates
5 g fiber
16 g protein
15 g fat
3 g saturated fat

Mediterranean Turkey Wrap

Prep Time: 2 minutes, **Total Time:** 10 minutes

Try this Mediterranean turkey wrap for a zesty, mid-day pick-me-up.

Ingredients:

- 1 La Tortilla Factory 100% Whole Wheat 100 Calorie Tortilla
- 2 tbsps roasted red pepper hummus
- 2 oz 98% fat-free deli turkey (usually 3-4 slices or 56 grams)
- ½ cup alfalfa sprouts
- ½ cup fresh baby spinach
- ⅛ cup Athenos Reduced-Fat Feta Cheese
- 2 fresh basil leaves, shredded
- 4 cherry tomatoes, sliced in half

Nutrition Information:
282 calories
34 g carbohydrates
12 g fiber
23 g protein
8 g fat
1 g saturated fat

Directions:

1. Spread hummus in middle of tortilla wrap and place turkey on top.
2. Cover with sprouts, spinach, feta, basil, and cherry tomatoes.
3. Roll up tortilla and enjoy.

Did You Know?
The health benefits of a Mediterranean-based diet are well known, with hummus among one of the top contributors. Hummus contains chickpeas, which are a great source of soluble fiber and help to lower cholesterol. Try substituting it for mayonnaise in sandwiches, for cream cheese on bagels, or as a dip with fresh vegetables.

Sweet Potato Panini with Strawberry Spinach Salad

Prep Time: 3 minutes, **Total Time:** 11 minutes

This sandwich contains the perfect combo of sweet and savory!

Directions:

1. Heat frying pan on medium heat.

2. While pan is heating, spread sandwich thins with hummus (1 tbsp on each side) and top with 7-8 spinach leaves, sprouts, and avocado.

3. Spray heated pan lightly with cooking spray, and place the 4 sweet potato slices in pan. Spray tops of slices lightly with cooking spray. Grill for 3 minutes on each side, or until soft.

4. While sweet potato slices are cooking, plate 1 cup of spinach and top with strawberries, walnuts, and light vinaigrette.

5. Remove sweet potato from pan, sprinkle lightly with sea salt and pepper, and place on sandwich. Serve toasted if preferred.

Ingredients:

- ¼ large sweet potato cut into 4, ¼-inch discs
- 2 tbsps red pepper hummus
- 1 sandwich thin
- ½ cup alfalfa sprouts
- 7-8 baby spinach leaves
- Salt and pepper

Salad:

- 1 cup baby spinach
- 3 strawberries, sliced
- 1 tsp crushed walnuts
- 1 tbsp light balsamic vinaigrette (try Newman's Own Organic Light Balsamic Dressing at only 23 calories per tbsp)

Nutrition Information:

366 calories
44 g carbohydrates
15 g fiber
12 g protein
19 g fat
2 g saturated fat

Crispy Club Sandwich

Prep Time: 6 minutes, **Total Time:** 11 minutes

Thoughts of restaurant style club sandwiches may send shivers up and down your spine (calories and fat–oh my!), but this version is low in both, and is also a good source of vitamin C.

Ingredients:

- 2 slices whole wheat bread, toasted
- 2 slices Jennie-O's Extra Lean Turkey Bacon, cooked
- 2 oz 98% fat-free deli turkey
- 2 slices of tomato
- 2 leaves of romaine lettuce
- 2 tsps fat-free mayonnaise

Directions:

1. Spread each slice of bread with 1 tsp of mayonnaise.

2. Top one slice with turkey, bacon, tomato, and lettuce.

3. Close sandwich and serve.

Did You Know?

The average club sandwich can run up to 700 calories and 30-40 grams of fat! Be wary of sandwiches packed with mayo, as their calories and fat can be off the charts, and way out of your calorie budget for the day. This sandwich swap is a good alternative to the traditional restaurant club.

Nutrition Information:

279 calories
32 g carbohydrates
6 g fiber
26 g protein
5 g fat
1 g saturated fat

Turkey-Bacon Melt

Prep Time: 7 minutes, Total Time: 12 minutes

The name of this recipe may make you think of fat, fat, and more fat, but this low-cal spin will change your mind. It's low in saturated fat, but still packed with cheesy, gooey flavor.

Directions:

1. Spread each slice of bread with 1 tsp of mayonnaise.

2. Top one slice with turkey, bacon, and tomato. Top other slice with cheese and the sprinkling of Italian seasoning, and close the sandwich.

3. Heat frying pan on medium heat. Spray lightly with cooking spray.

4. Place sandwich in pan, cheese side down, cooking for 2 minutes. Flip and cook an additional 1-2 minutes, until bread is toasted and cheese is melted.

Ingredients:

- 2 slices whole wheat bread
- 2 slices Jennie-O's Extra Lean Turkey Bacon, cooked
- 2 oz 98% fat-free deli turkey
- 1 slice of fat-free cheddar cheese
- ¼ tsp Italian spice blend
- 2 tsps fat-free mayonnaise
- 2 slices of tomato
- Olive oil cooking spray

Nutrition Information:

278 calories
32 g carbohydrates
5 g fiber
27 g protein
4 g fat
1 g saturated fat

Avocado Bean Sandwich

Prep Time: 8 minutes, **Total Time:** 10 minutes

A great option for vegetarians, this sandwich is flavorful and full of heart-healthy fats and fiber.

Ingredients:

- 1 Arnold Select 100% Whole Wheat Sandwich Thin
- ½ cup canned white beans, rinsed to remove excess sodium
- ½ tsp olive oil
- ⅛ tsp salt
- ⅛ tsp ground black pepper
- 3 thin slices of red onion
- 4 cucumber slices, with peel
- ½ cup alfalfa sprouts
- ½ avocado, pitted and sliced

Directions:

1. In a small bowl, mash together beans, olive oil, salt, and pepper.

2. Spread mixture onto sandwich thin.
   Top with red onion, cucumber, alfalfa sprouts, and avocado.

3. Close sandwich and serve.

Did You Know?
Sometimes the time of day is enough encouragement to eat a meal, despite a lack of actual physical hunger. But don't eat a big meal just because it's lunch time. Instead, learn to listen to your body. A quick snack may be all you need.

Nutrition Information:
387 calories
55 g carbohydrates
17 g fiber
17 g protein
14 g fat
2 g saturated fat

Halibut Salad

Prep Time: 15 minutes, **Total Time:** 20 minutes

This salad is a refreshingly low-calorie lunch-time treat, and is a great way to incorporate more fish into your diet. Try this with a number of different fish fillets (salmon, tuna, tilapia, etc.).

Directions:

1. Season fish with salt and pepper to taste, and simmer in ½ inch of water on medium-high heat to cook, about 6-8 minutes.

2. Set fish aside to cool, and flake into large pieces.

3. Plate salad greens and top with halibut pieces, chickpeas, avocado, and red onion.

4. In a small bowl or dressing container, thoroughly mix olive oil, lemon juice, mustard, cilantro, salt, and pepper.

5. Drizzle salad with vinaigrette and serve.

Nutrition Information:
292 calories
21 g carbohydrates
7 g fiber, 24 g protein
13 g fat
2 g saturated fat

Ingredients:

- 3-oz piece of halibut
- Salt and pepper to taste
- 2 cups mixed salad greens
- ¼ cup canned chickpeas, rinsed to remove excess sodium
- ¼ avocado, peeled and pitted
- 3 slices of red onion

Vinaigrette:

- 1 tbsp olive oil
- ½ tsp lemon juice
- ½ tsp Dijon mustard
- ½ tbsp fresh chopped cilantro
- ⅛ tsp salt
- ⅛ ground black pepper

LUNCH

Tarragon-Lime Chicken and Bacon Wrap

Prep Time: 8 minutes, Total Time: 12 minutes

This zesty chicken wrap is a great source of fiber and protein, and is packed with vitamins A, B6, and K. It's also low in saturated fat, making it a heart-healthy and low-calorie lunch.

Ingredients:

- 1 La Tortilla Factory 100% Whole Wheat 100 Calorie Tortilla
- 2 tbsps fat-free mayonnaise
- ½ tsp lemon juice
- ¼ tsp dried tarragon
- ½ cup shredded lettuce
- ½ cup chopped tomato
- 1 slice Jennie-O's extra lean turkey bacon, cooked
- 4 oz diced chicken breast, skinless boneless, cooked (about ½ cup)

Nutrition Information:
284 calories
32 g carbohydrates
10 g fiber
35 g protein
4 g fat
1 g saturated fat

Directions:

1. In a small dish, mix mayonnaise, tarragon, and lemon juice.

2. Spread mayonnaise mixture down the middle of tortilla wrap, and top with chicken, lettuce, and tomato. Crumble bacon over top.

3. Roll up tortilla and enjoy.

Did You Know?
The name "tarragon" comes from the French word estragon, which means "little dragon." Some think the herb was given this name for its supposed ability to cure venomous reptile bites. Tarragon has a pleasant licorice-like aroma with a bittersweet taste, and is great paired with chicken, fish, egg, or vegetable dishes.

Chicken Shawarma

Prep Time: 20 minutes, Total Time: 40 minutes

This middle-eastern dish makes a tasty, flavor-packed lunch.

Directions:

1. Heat frying pan on medium heat.

2. While pan heats up, mix lemon juice, curry powder, olive oil, salt cumin, and garlic.

3. Toss chicken in mixture to coat. Refrigerate for 20 minutes to let marinate.

4. Prepare sauce by mixing yogurt, tahini, lemon juice, garlic, and dash of salt.

5. Remove chicken from refrigerator and spray frying pan lightly with olive oil cooking spray. Place chicken in pan. Cook until done, turning occasionally. Remove chicken from pan when finished.

6. Re-spray frying pan with cooking oil. Place pitas in pan and grill each side lightly, about 1 minute per side.

7. Place grilled pita on plate, top with grilled chicken, lettuce, tomato, and sauce.

Ingredients:

- 1 Joseph's Flax, Oat Bran & Whole Wheat Pita
- ¼ cup shredded romaine lettuce
- 2 tomato slices
- Olive oil cooking spray
- 4 oz chicken breast, skinless, boneless, cut into strips
- ½ tbsp lemon juice
- ¼ tsp curry powder
- ½ tsp olive oil
- ⅛ tsp salt
- ⅛ tsp ground cumin
- ¾ tsp of minced garlic

Sauce:

- 2 tbsps non-fat, plain Greek yogurt
- ½ tbsp tahini
- ½ tsp lemon juice
- ¼ tsp minced garlic
- Dash of salt

Nutrition Information:

282 calories, 15 g carbohydrates, 5 g fiber, 37 g protein, 10 g fat, 1 g saturated fat

Toasted Chipotle Tuna Sandwich

Prep Time: 5 minutes, **Total Time:** 11 minutes

Subbing Greek yogurt for mayo in your tuna sandwich not only cuts back on fat and calories, but also ups the flavor factor and protein power.

Ingredients:

- 1 sandwich thin
- 1 leaf of romaine lettuce
- 1-2 tomato slices
- 1 can of chunk light albacore tuna, in water
- ½ stick of celery, diced
- 1 tbsp of non-fat plain Greek yogurt
- ¼ tsp of ground black pepper
- ⅛ tsp lemon juice
- 2 ½ tsps honey Dijon mustard
- ¼ tsp chipotle chile pepper seasoning

Directions:

1. Place lettuce and tomato on sandwich thin.

2. In a small bowl, mix rest of ingredients together.

3. Top sandwich with tuna mixture, close, and place in toaster oven until bread is toasted.

Did You Know?

The United States uses over 31% of the total amount of tuna caught in the world? Most of the tuna we consume is canned, which can come packed in either water or oil. Both types can fit into a healthy diet, though tuna packed in water is slightly lower in calories (109 calories versus 158 for a 3-ounce serving).

Nutrition Information:

334 calories
26 g carbohydrates
6 g fiber
49 g protein
2 g fat
0 g saturated fat

Spinach Flatbread Pizza

Prep Time: 0 minutes, **Total Time:** 10 minutes

Let this flatbread pizza take you away from your kitchen and back to rustic Italy—sans the calories.

Directions:

1. Preheat oven to 425°F.
2. Spray baking sheet lightly with cooking spray.
3. Place tortilla on baking sheet and spread with tomato sauce, leaving a small ring on outer edges as a crust.
4. Top with spinach, mushrooms, and mozzarella.
5. Bake pizza for 10 minutes, or until crust turns golden brown.

Ingredients:

- 1 La Tortilla Factory 100% Whole Wheat 100 Calorie Tortilla
- ¼ cup tomato sauce
- ½ cup shredded, low-fat mozzarella cheese
- ½ cup frozen spinach, thawed and drained
- ½ cup chopped, white mushrooms

Did You Know?

You can now buy mushrooms fortified with vitamin D? Three-quarters of U.S. teens and adults are deficient in vitamin D, which is usually only found in animal foods or received from sun exposure.

Nutrition Information:

315 calories
37 g carbohydrates
12 g fiber
24 g protein
14 g fat
6 g saturated fat

Chilled Shrimp Salad

Prep Time: 15 minutes, **Total Time:** 20 minutes

This shrimp salad is a delicious and simple addition to your meal plan for the day. Topped with flavor-bursting feta cheese and cilantro, it's sure to lighten up your plate.

Ingredients:

- 2 cups mixed salad greens
- 3 ½ oz cooked and peeled shrimp
- ¼ cup chopped cucumber
- ¼ cup diced tomato
- ¼ cup canned chickpeas, rinsed to remove excess sodium
- 2 tbsps Athenos Reduced Fat Feta Cheese
- 2 tsps olive oil
- ½ tsp cilantro
- ½ tbsp red wine vinegar
- Dash of salt and pepper to taste

Directions:

1. Toss all ingredients together in a small bowl. Serve chilled.

Did You Know?

Four ounces of shrimp provides almost half the daily requirement of vitamin D, also known as the "sunshine vitamin." Vitamin D helps us build strong bones, maintain a healthy immune system, and may also lower the risk of certain conditions, like type 2 diabetes and high blood pressure.

Nutrition Information:

387 calories
17 g carbohydrates
6 g fiber, 39 g protein
16 g fat, 4 g saturated fat

Greek Salad Pita

Prep Time: 6 minutes, **Total Time:** 8 minutes

This pita is the perfect way to enjoy your Greek salad on the go, and it's packed full of fiber to help you stay full until dinner.

Directions:

1. In a small bowl, mix lettuce, feta cheese, cherry tomatoes, red onion, lemon juice, and Parmesan cheese.

2. Cut opening in pita, fill with salad mixture, and serve.

Ingredients:

- 1 Joseph's Flax, Oat Bran & Whole Wheat Pita
- 1 ½ cups shredded romaine lettuce
- ⅛ cup Athenos Reduced-Fat Feta Cheese
- 6 cherry tomatoes, sliced in half
- ⅛ cup chopped red onion
- 1 tbsp fat-free Parmesan cheese
- 1 tbsp lemon juice

Did You Know?

The term "Greek salad" is used in North America to refer to a salad with Greek-inspired ingredients, dressed with oil and vinegar. The most standard elements are lettuce, tomatoes, feta cheese, and olives, with other ingredients sometimes varying on location. In Detroit, Michigan, for example, a "Greek salad" also includes beets, and in Tampa Bay, Florida, it often includes potato salad.

Nutrition Information:
293 calories
29 g carbohydrates
8 g fiber
26 g protein
8 g fat
3 g saturated fat

Fresh Tarragon-Chicken Potato Chicken Salad

Prep Time: 15 minutes, **Total Time:** 20 minutes

This chicken salad is low in saturated fat, but packed with protein, vitamins, minerals, and flavor. Go ahead and serve it cold or warm—it's delicious either way!

Ingredients:

- 4 oz cooked, cubed chicken breast (about ½ cup)
- 1 cup baby spinach leaves
- ½ cup chopped snap peas
- 1 small, red skin potato, chopped
- ¼ cup chopped red bell pepper
- 2 tbsps chopped red onion
- ½ tbsp olive oil
- ½ tbsp white wine vinegar
- ¾ tsp lemon juice
- ¾ tsp Dijon mustard
- ¼ tsp dried tarragon
- ¼ tsp salt
- ⅛ tsp ground black pepper
- ¼ tsp minced garlic

Directions:

1. Place potato and snap peas in a microwave safe bowl. Pour in 1 tbsp of water, cover partially, and microwave on high for 4-5 minutes, or until tender.

2. Place spinach leaves, potato, and snap peas in a small salad bowl. Top with chicken, bell pepper, and onion.

3. In a small bowl or dressing container, thoroughly mix olive oil, white wine vinegar, lemon juice, mustard, tarragon, salt, pepper, and garlic.

4. Top chicken salad with dressing, toss to coat, and serve.

Nutrition Information:
361 calories
38 g carbohydrates
6 g fiber
32 g protein
9 g fat, 1 g saturated fat

Chicken Waldorf Salad

Prep Time: 15 minutes, **Total Time:** 20 minutes

This salad is everything you could ask for in a lunch: sweet, crunchy, low in calories, and bursting at the seams with flavor. Plus, it's loaded with 22 grams of satiating protein!

Directions:

1. Toss apple slices with lemon juice.

2. Toss remaining ingredients and apple slices in a salad bowl.

3. Drizzle raspberry vinaigrette over salad. Serve and enjoy.

Did You Know?

Tart cherries, whether enjoyed dried or frozen, have among the highest levels of disease-fighting antioxidants, when compared with other fruits. They also contain other important nutrients like beta-carotene (19 times more than blueberries or strawberries), Vitamin C, magnesium, potassium, iron, folate, and fiber.

Ingredients:

- 3 oz chicken breast, boneless, skinless, diced (cooked)
- 2 cups mixed salad greens
- ¼ tsp lemon juice
- ½ cup chopped Gala apples
- ¼ cup green grapes, halved
- 2 tbsps chopped celery
- 2 tbsps chopped walnuts
- 2 tbsps dried cherries
- ¼ of 1 red onion, thinly sliced
- 2 tbsps reduced-fat raspberry vinaigrette

Nutrition Information:

305 calories
37 g carbohydrates
4 g fiber
22 g protein
8 g fat, 1 g saturated fat

Tomato and Goat Cheese Mini Pizzas

Prep Time: 10 minutes, **Total Time:** 15 minutes

This colorful spin on pizza is a quick and easy lunch option. It's also full of calcium and bursting with flavor.

Ingredients:

- 1 whole wheat English muffin
- 1 oz crumbled goat cheese
- ¼ cup reduced-fat mozzarella cheese
- ¼ tsp minced garlic
- ¼ cup chopped cherry tomatoes

Directions:

1. Cut English muffin in half.
2. Rub each half of the muffin with garlic.
3. Sprinkle with tomato and cheeses.
4. Broil in conventional or toaster oven until cheese is melted. Serve and enjoy.

Did You Know?

Goat cheese is one of the earliest made dairy products, and comes in many shapes and flavors: cone-shaped, disc, wheel, strong and pungent, delicate, and mild—the list is endless. Compared with cheese from a cow, goat cheese is lower in fat, calories, and cholesterol, and provides more calcium than cream cheese!

Nutrition Information:

338 calories
30 g carbohydrates
5 g fiber, 22 g protein
16 g fat
10 g saturated fat

Turkey Stuffed Bell Pepper

Prep Time: 30 minutes, **Total Time:** 1 hour & 30 minutes

This flavorful stuffed pepper is rich in B vitamins, potassium, vitamin C, and lean protein. Try making a larger batch of these for a quick and easy meal every night of the week.

Directions:

1. Preheat oven to 350°F.

2. In a skillet over medium-high heat, cook ground turkey, thoroughly browning.

3. Cut off top stem part of bell pepper, removing seeds and membranes.

4. In a small bowl, mix browned turkey, cooked rice, tomato sauce, Worcestershire sauce, garlic, onion powder, onion, and salt and pepper. Spoon mixture into hollowed bell pepper.

5. Mix topping ingredients (Italian seasoning and 1/8 cup of tomato sauce) and pour over stuffed pepper.

6. Bake for 45 minutes to 1 hour in the oven, or until pepper is tender. Marinate occasionally with extra tomato sauce if desired.

Ingredients:

- 3 oz extra lean ground turkey, raw
- ¼ cup cooked brown rice
- 2 ½ tbsps water
- 1 green bell pepper
- ½ cup tomato sauce
- ½ tsp Worcestershire sauce
- ⅛ tsp minced garlic
- ⅛ tsp onion powder
- ¼ of 1 small white onion, diced
- Dash of salt and pepper

Topping:

- ⅛ tsp Italian seasoning
- ⅛ cup tomato sauce

Nutrition Information:
255 calories,
28 g carbohydrates
6 g fiber, 19 g protein
8 g fat, 2 g saturated fat

Eggplant Parmesan

Prep Time: 30 minutes, **Total Time:** 1 hour

This dish may taste and smell like comfort food, but the calorie-count says otherwise.

Ingredients:

- 1 slice of eggplant, about ¾ inch thick
- ½ tsp salt 1 tbsp olive oil
- 2 tbsps fat-free ricotta cheese
- 2 tbsps reduced-fat mozzarella cheese
- 1 tbsp fat-free Parmesan cheese
- ⅛ cup egg substitutes (like Egg Beaters)
- 1 tsp dried basil
- ½ cup pasta sauce

Nutrition Information:

321 calories
28 g carbohydrates
6 g fiber
15 g protein
17 g fat
4 g saturated fat

Directions:

1. Preheat oven to 350°F.

2. Sprinkle both sides of eggplant with salt, and let it sweat in a colander in the sink for 20-30 minutes.

3. While eggplant sweats, in a small bowl, mix ricotta, mozzarella, Parmesan cheese, egg, and dried basil. Set aside.

4. Heat frying pan on medium-high heat. Heat olive oil in pan.

5. Rinse the eggplant to remove salt, and transfer eggplant to pan. Brown each side of eggplant.

6. Pour pasta sauce into a small baking dish. Transfer eggplant slice on top of pasta sauce.

7. Top eggplant slice with cheese mixture.

8. Bake 30-45 minutes or until cheese bubbles.

Lemon-Pepper Chicken and Rice

Prep Time: 5 minutes, **Total Time:** 8-10 hours

Throw these ingredients together in the morning, and let it cook while you're away at work for a delicious and simple meal when you walk through the door.

Directions:

1. Combine rice, water, and bouillon cube in crock pot.

2. Rub chicken breast with lemon peel, pepper, and sage, and place on top of rice. Sprinkle with minced garlic.

3. Let simmer for 8-10 hours, or until rice is fully cooked and water has been absorbed.

4. 10 minutes before serving, add frozen broccoli florets and sprinkle with salt and pepper. Let cook for 10 minutes to steam broccoli, then serve.

Ingredients:

- 3 oz chicken breast (raw)
- ¼ tsp lemon peel
- ¼ tsp ground black pepper
- ¼ tsp sage
- ½ tsp minced garlic
- ¼ cup brown rice, uncooked
- ½ bouillon cube
- ½ cup of water
- 1 cup of frozen broccoli florets
- Dash of salt and pepper

Nutrition Information:
315 calories
45 g carbohydrates
7 g fiber
28 g protein
3 g fat
1 g saturated fat

Spice Rubbed Salmon with Citrus Asparagus and Wild Rice

Prep Time: 10 minutes, **Total Time:** 30 minutes

Nutritious, fiber-packed, and tasty, this meal is sure to please!

Ingredients:

- Olive oil cooking spray
- ¼ white onion, sliced
- 7 asparagus spears (cut in half)
- 1 tsp lemon juice
- ½ tsp sea salt
- ⅛ tsp ground pepper
- ⅛ tsp ground coriander
- ¼ tsp paprika
- ¼ tsp ground cumin
- ½ cup Uncle Ben's 90 Second Ready Whole Grain Medley Brown and Wild Rice

Nutrition Information:

329 calories
30 g carbohydrates,
5 g fiber
23 g protein
14 g fat
3 g saturated fat

Directions:

1. Preheat oven to 400°F.

2. Lightly coat 9x13 pan with cooking spray and fill with onion slices. Lay asparagus spears down on top of onions and sprinkle them with the lemon juice. Spray both onions and asparagus lightly with olive oil spray.

3. Combine salt, pepper, coriander, paprika, and cumin in a small bowl. Rub mixture on salmon filet until well covered. Place salmon filet in pan on top of asparagus bed. Place pan in oven and bake for 20 minutes.

4. When salmon is close to being done, prepare rice according to directions. Plate ½ cup of rice, storing rest in refrigerator.

5. Remove pan from oven, place onions, asparagus, and salmon on top of rice, and enjoy!

Vegetarian Chili

Prep Time: 10 minutes, Total Time: 6-8 hours

The fabulous thing about this recipe is that it's minimal work with maximum flavor. Try throwing the ingredients in your crock pot in the morning for a delicious hot meal you get home!

Directions:

1. Combine all ingredients in small crock pot and let simmer for 6-8 hours.* Makes 2 servings.

   *Alternatively you can combine ingredients in a saucepan and let simmer for 30 minutes on low heat before serving.

Ingredients:

- 1 can of spicy chili beans
- 8 oz of salsa
- 8 ¾-oz can of whole kernel corn

Did You Know?

Texas-style chili contains no beans, and is often made with no other vegetables besides chili peppers. White chili is made using great northern beans and turkey meat or chicken breast. And vegetarian chili, also known as chili sin carne (chili without meat), leaves meat out entirely.

Nutrition Information:

1 serving of chili:
226 calories
43 g carbohydrates
11 g fiber
10 g protein
2 g fat
0 g saturated fat

Baked Spaghetti Pie

Prep Time: 13 minutes, **Total Time:** 40 minutes

Bored with plain spaghetti? Mix it up with this quick and easy spaghetti pie—a low-calorie twist on an Italian classic.

Ingredients:

- ¾ cup cooked spaghetti noodles
- ¼ cup Egg Beaters
- ¼ tsp oregano leaves
- ¼ tsp ground pepper
- ⅛ cup fat-free ricotta cheese
- 2 tbsps fat-free Parmesan cheese
- ⅓ cup marinara sauce
- Olive oil cooking spray

Directions:

1. Preheat oven to 350°F.

2. Stir Egg Beaters, Parmesan cheese, oregano, and black pepper in with cooked spaghetti noodles.

3. Spray an oven-safe ramekin or small, single serving casserole bowl with cooking spray.

4. Place noodles in bowl and top with ricotta cheese, followed by marinara sauce. Bake for 20 minutes.

5. Remove from oven and let cool for 7 minutes before serving.

Nutrition Information:
362 calories
54 g carbohydrates
8 g fiber
27 g protein
4 g fat
2 g saturated fat

Spicy Chipotle Chicken

Prep Time: 3 minutes, **Total Time:** 5-6 hours

This slow-cooked chicken meal is low in saturated fat, a good source of fiber, and filled with protein. Plus, it's packed with flavors that will make your taste buds curl.

Directions:

1. Place chicken breast in bottom of a crock pot and surround with salsa.

2. Sprinkle chicken with cumin, chipotle chile pepper, chili powder, and minced garlic.

3. Top with black beans.

4. Let simmer for 5-6 hours, or until chicken is thoroughly cooked.

5. 10 minutes before serving, add bell pepper mix. Let cook until bell peppers are thoroughly cooked, and serve.

Ingredients:

- 3 oz skinless, boneless chicken breast (raw)
- ⅛ cup salsa
- ¼ tsp ground cumin
- ¼ tsp chipotle chile pepper
- ⅛ tsp chili powder
- 1 clove of minced garlic
- ¼, 15 ½-oz can black beans (rinsed to remove excess sodium)
- 1 cup frozen bell pepper mix

Nutrition Information:

278 calories
34 g carbohydrates
11 g fiber
31 g protein
2 g fat
0 g saturated fat

Black Pepper Tuna With Artichokes

Prep Time: 10 minutes, **Total Time:** 20 minutes

This dish provides winning flavor that's easy on your waistline.

Ingredients:

- ¾ cup frozen artichoke hearts, thawed
- 3 tbsps diced, canned tomatoes
- 1 ½ tsps olive oil
- 1 clove minced garlic
- ½ tbsp lemon juice
- ¼ tsp ground thyme
- 6 oz Ahi tuna steak, raw
- ½ cup brown rice, cooked (recommended: 90 second rice)
- Dash of salt and pepper
- Olive oil cooking spray

Nutrition Information:

395 calories
32 g carbohydrates
5 g fiber
45 g protein
9 g fat
2 g saturated fat

Directions:

1. Prepare brown rice according to directions, plate ½ cup and set aside.

2. Place fry pan on burner on medium heat. Let heat thoroughly, and spritz lightly with olive oil spray.

3. While burner heats, combine artichoke hearts, tomatoes, olive oil, garlic, lemon juice, and thyme in a frying pan and stir over medium heat.

4. Sprinkle each side of tuna steak lightly with salt and pepper.

5. Once pan is heated, place tuna steak in pan, searing for 1 minute on each side.

6. While tuna is cooking, continue to stir artichoke and tomato mixture. Sprinkle with a dash of salt and pepper.

7. Set tuna on top of rice.

8. Transfer artichoke and tomato mixture from pan onto tuna and rice.

Black Bean Soup

Prep Time: 2 minutes, **Total Time:** 18 minutes

Homemade soup is the perfect way to warm up on a chilly day. This comfort-food recipe is packed full of nutrient-rich beans, fiber, and protein.

Directions:

1. Heat olive oil over medium heat in a saucepan, adding ⅓ cup salsa and cooking for 2-3 minutes.

2. Add black beans, refried beans, and vegetable broth, bringing to a boil. Reduce heat and simmer for 5 minutes.

3. Pour soup into a bowl and top with sour cream, 1 tbsp of salsa, and cilantro. Serve.

Did You Know?
Research has shown that draining and rinsing your canned beans can reduce sodium by up to 40%! The USDA's Dietary Guidelines recommends the general U.S. population limit their sodium intake to less than about a teaspoon.

Ingredients:

Soup:
- ¼ tsp olive oil
- ⅓ cup salsa
- ½ cup canned black beans, rinsed to remove excess sodium
- ½ cup fat-free refried beans
- ½ cup low-sodium vegetable broth

Topping:
- 1 tbsp fat-free sour cream
- 1 tbsp salsa
- 1 tbsp freshly chopped cilantro

Nutrition Information:
263 calories
46 g carbohydrates
14 g fiber
16 g protein
2 g fat
0 g saturated fat

White Bean Chicken and Tomatoes

Prep Time: 5 minutes, **Total Time:** 30 minutes

You won't be disappointed as the aroma of thyme and oregano fill your kitchen from this simple and delicious recipe.

Ingredients:

- 3 oz boneless, skinless, chicken breast (raw)
- ¾ cup white beans, rinsed to remove excess sodium
- ½ cup cherry tomatoes, cut in half
- 1 tsp thyme
- 1 tsp oregano
- ½ clove minced garlic
- ⅛ tsp crushed red pepper
- 1 ½ tsp olive oil
- ⅛ tsp salt
- ⅛ tsp ground black pepper

Directions:

1. Preheat oven to 425°F.

2. Combine beans, tomatoes, thyme, oregano, minced garlic, red pepper, 1 tsp olive oil, salt, and pepper in a small baking dish.

3. Place chicken breast on top of bean mixture, and rub with remaining ½ tsp olive oil. Season lightly with dash of salt and pepper.

4. Bake dish until chicken is cooked thoroughly, about 25-30 minutes.

Nutrition Information:

352 calories
37 g carbohydrates
10 g fiber
33 g protein
8 g fat
1 g saturated fat

Pan Seared Tilapia and Clementine Salad

Prep Time: 6 minutes, **Total Time:** 15 minutes

This fish dish is packed with protein, spices, and vitamins, and is sure to delight even the most discriminating taste-buds.

Directions:

1. Heat frying pan on medium-high heat until hot. Spray lightly with olive oil cooking spray.

2. Season tilapia fillet with salt and pepper, and add to pan.

3. Cook 1-2 minutes on each side, or until cooked through, and easily flakes. Transfer to plate.

4. In a small container with a lid, mix olive oil, lime juice, ginger, honey, salt, and red pepper.

5. Plate salad greens and top with Clementine orange slices. Plate fish with salad.

6. Drizzle fish and salad with dressing, and serve.

Ingredients:

Soup:

- 3 oz fillet of tilapia, raw
- Dash of salt and ground black pepper
- 1 Clementine orange, peeled, and sectioned
- 1 cup mixed salad greens
- Olive oil cooking spray

Topping:

- 1 tbsp olive oil
- ½ tbsp lime juice
- ½ tsp crushed ginger
- ½ tsp honey
- ⅛ tsp salt
- Dash of crushed red pepper

Nutrition Information:
283 calories
14 g carbohydrates
2 g fiber
23 g protein
16 g fat
3 g saturated fat

Penne Pasta e Fagioli

Prep Time: 15 minutes, **Total Time:** 20 minutes

Pasta e fagioli means "pasta and beans" in Italian. It may sound boring, but this dish is anything but. The hearty beans and bright tomatoes will make you feel like you're sitting in Venice!

Ingredients:

- 1 cup cooked, whole wheat penne pasta noodles
- ½ tsp olive oil
- 1 clove garlic, minced
- ⅓ cup canned white beans, rinsed to remove excess sodium
- ½ cup diced tomato
- 1 tbsp fat-free Parmesan cheese
- ½ tsp oregano
- Salt and pepper to taste

Directions:

1. Heat frying pan on medium heat and combine olive oil, tomato, garlic, and beans.

2. When bean mixture is thoroughly heated, remove from frying pan and add to small bowl with cooked penne pasta noodles.

3. Add Parmesan cheese and oregano, stir, and serve.

Did You Know?

Garlic has been used for both culinary and medicinal purposes throughout the years, and was even mentioned in the Bible. Crushing or cutting garlic releases a compound called allicin, which research has shown may aid in heart health.

Nutrition Information:

375 calories
66 g carbohydrates
11 g fiber
19 g protein
5 g fat
1 g saturated fat

Sweet & Savory Meatless Tacos

Prep Time: 15 minutes, **Total Time:** 20 minutes

Meatless taco night doesn't have to mean just beans—delicious meatless-meat crumbles are the perfect vegetarian substitution. And the mango salsa on these tacos packs a tasty, sweet tang.

Directions:

1. Heat frying pan on medium-high heat. Pour in frozen Morningstar crumbles, water, and taco seasoning. Heat, stirring until heated thoroughly.

2. Split taco meat evenly between tortillas.

3. Top each taco with 2 tbsps of salsa, 2 tbsps sour cream, ½ cup lettuce, and ¼ cup diced tomatoes.

4. Roll and serve.

Ingredients:

- 2 La Tortilla Factory 100% Whole Wheat 50 Calorie Tortillas
- 1 cup frozen Morning-star Farms Meal Starters Grillers Recipe Crumbles
- ½ packet of taco seasoning
- ⅓ cup of water
- 4 tbsps Newman's Own Mango Salsa
- 4 tbsps fat-free sour cream
- 1 cup shredded romaine lettuce
- ½ cup diced tomatoes

Nutrition Information:

323 calories
57 g carbohydrates
18 g fiber
24 g protein
5 g fat
0 g saturated fat

DINNER

Garlic & Lemon Shrimp and Couscous

Prep Time: 15 minutes, **Total Time:** 25 minutes

The couscous in this dish brings a hint of exotic flavor. It's still super easy to prepare, and is a great source of filling fiber and protein.

Ingredients:

- ⅓ cup couscous, cooked
- ½ tbsp butter
- ½ clove minced garlic
- 4 oz shrimp, cooked, peeled, and deveined
- ½ cup canned white beans, rinsed to remove excess sodium
- ½ tbsp lemon juice
- 1 tbsp parsley
- ⅛ tsp salt
- ⅛ tsp pepper

Directions:

1. Cook couscous according to package directions. Set aside ⅓ for meal, store rest in refrigerator.

2. Heat butter in frying pan on medium heat.

3. Add garlic and shrimp, and heat for about 3-4 minutes, or until thoroughly heated through.

4. Stir in beans, lemon juice, parsley, salt, and pepper.

5. Cook until thoroughly heated. Serve shrimp mixture over couscous.

Nutrition Information:
345 calories
36 g carbohydrates
10 g fiber
32 g protein
7 g fat
2 g saturated fat

20 Healthy Snacks Under 200 Calories

1. 2 tbsps peanut butter
   15 whole wheat crackers

2. Baby carrots, red pepper
   2 tbsps hummus

3. Laughing Cow Light Cheese
   15 whole wheat crackers

4. Sliced papaya with
   lime juice

5. Low-fat string cheese
   Apple or pear

6. Can of tuna
   Sliced black olives
   Lemon juice

7. 1 tbsp peanut butter
   Apple slices

8. 2 slices of turkey
   1 slice of Swiss cheese
   Mustard for dipping

9. Sliced tomato
   Sliced mozzarella
   Drizzle of olive oil

10. 1 ounce raspberries
    Cottage cheese

11. Multi-grain pita
    2 tbsps hummus

12. 4 cups light popcorn
    Sprinkle of Parmesan
    cheese

13. 1 cup raspberries
    20-25 almonds

14. 5 strawberries
    Cool Whip Light

15. 1 tbsp almond butter
    Apple slices

16. 2 slices of turkey
    Small multi-grain tortilla
    Salsa

17. ½ cup cottage cheese
    20-25 almonds

18. 5-10 olives
    1 cup unshelled
    edamame

19. Cottage cheese
    Canned pineapple, drained

20. 1 cup sugar snap peas
    Tossed with
    2 tbsps Parmesan

Notes:

_____

_____

_____

_____

_____

_____

_____

_____

_____

_____

_____

_____

_____

_____

_____

_____

_____

_____

_____

_____

## Chapter 13

How to Use the Journal Pages

These journal pages are an instrumental part of your success losing weight and belly fat in 30 days. They help you monitor your weight, calorie intake, and calories burned through exercise. And the best way to create a significant calorie deficit per day is to plan ahead and create a calorie "budget," as well as to determine how much exercise you need to burn additional calories. Anticipating how many calories you can "spend" takes the guesswork out of cooking and ordering from restaurant menus. You can track how well you follow your fitness goals by recording exactly how many calories you consume and burn on a daily basis with these journal pages.

The journal pages also give you clues about how food, exercise, and hydration factor into your mood and energy levels. You may find fascinating correlations between what you're eating and how great or lousy you're feeling. Plus, nothing is a better motivator for exercise than realizing how much energy you have throughout the day when you've hit the gym or gone for a bike ride.

Another great benefit of a diet and fitness journal is that it keeps you accountable. It's easy to let a 150-calorie cookie slip your mind, but those little white lies are much more difficult when you're recording everything in a journal. You've likely put on extra weight by not holding yourself accountable in the past. This journal will help you break that bad habit. Use these journal pages to record everything you eat, drink, and do by way of exercise. It's the proven way to slim down faster!

Here is an explanation of the various components of the journal pages:

❶ DAILY NUTRITIONAL INTAKE: Record your daily intake of calories, fats, and carbs. Compare these totals to your nutritional intake goal from earlier in this book and see if you are meeting your targeted amounts. There is also an "Other" column that can be used to track intake of protein, fiber, sugar, sodium, or other nutrients if you have special dietary concerns, such as high blood pressure or diabetes.

❷ WATER INTAKE: Strive for at least eight 8-ounce glasses of water per day. Check off a box for each glass you drink. If you drink water on a regular basis, your metabolism works faster and better, and you'll have more energy.

❸ DAILY EXERCISE: Record all physical activity you perform. Be sure to jot down the time you spend and the number of calories you burn with each exercise. With time, you should see those numbers increase as your energy levels increase and as you gain more stamina.

❹ ENERGY LEVEL: Document your daily energy levels by rating your energy levels from low to high. Take note of how your energy correlates to the types of foods you have eaten that day. For example, if you notice that a little extra protein helps you get through your workout with more energy, incorporate lean meats in your diet. As you discover these relationships, make adjustments as needed to help you feel your best.

❺ CALORIE CALCULATOR: This formula helps you find your Daily Net Calorie Gain or Loss for each day. Start with your Total Calorie Intake for that day, and subtract the Total Calories Burned from physical activity to get your Net Calories. Then subtract your BMR (the number of calories your body burns at rest, calculated earlier in this book) to get your Daily Net Calorie Gain or Loss. Your goal is for this to be a negative number, meaning you created a calorie deficit, which is necessary to lose weight.

DATE: Feb. 2   **WEIGHT:** 197

❶ NUTRITIONAL INTAKE

🍎 FOOD/BEVERAGE	Qty.	Calories	Fat	Carbs	Other
Blueberry scone	1	400	17	55	5
Orange juice	12oz.	110	0	26	2
Bagel w/ turkey		490	4	70	30
American cheese	2	64	2	2	8
Baby carrots		100	0	24	3
Pepsi	12oz.	180	0	45	0
Apple slices + peanut butter		245	17	21	10
Salmon	8oz.	416	22	0	45
Wild Rice		166	2	34	7
Broccoli		54	1	12	2
DAILY INTAKE TOTALS:		2,225	65	289	112

❸ DAILY EXERCISE

❷ ☑ Water Intake
# of 8 oz. glasses

☑ ☑ ☑
☑ ☑ ☑
☑ ☑ ☐

❹ ENERGY LEVEL:
☑ low
☐ medium
☐ high

Activity	Hrs./Mins.	Cal. Burned
Playing basketball	60 mins	300
Jogging around my neighborhood	20 mins	205
Push-ups	10 mins	35
Pull-ups	5 mins	25
Stretching	10 mins	5
DAILY TOTALS:		570

❺ CALORIE CALCULATOR

2,225	−	570	=	1,655	−	1,979	=	−324
TOTAL CALORIE INTAKE		TOTAL CALORIES BURNED		NET CALORIES		BMR (Basal Metabolic Rate)		DAILY NET CALORIE GAIN OR LOSS

Notes:

Day 1

DATE: _____ WEIGHT: _____

NUTRITIONAL INTAKE

FOOD/BEVERAGE	Qty.	Calories	Fat	Carbs	Other
_____	_____				
_____	_____				
_____	_____				
_____	_____				
_____	_____				
_____	_____				
_____	_____				
_____	_____				
_____	_____				
_____	_____				
DAILY INTAKE TOTALS:					

DAILY EXERCISE

☑ **Water Intake**
# of 8 oz. glasses

◯◯◯
◯◯◯
◯◯◯

ENERGY LEVEL:

◯ low

◯ medium

◯ high

Activity	Hrs./Mins.	Cal. Burned
_____	_____	
_____	_____	
_____	_____	
_____	_____	
_____	_____	
DAILY TOTALS:		

CALORIE CALCULATOR

	−		=		−		=	
TOTAL CALORIE INTAKE		TOTAL CALORIES BURNED		NET CALORIES		BMR (Basal Metabolic Rate)		DAILY NET CALORIE GAIN OR LOSS

Day 2

DATE: _____ WEIGHT: _____

NUTRITIONAL INTAKE

FOOD/BEVERAGE	Qty.	Calories	Fat	Carbs	Other
DAILY INTAKE TOTALS:					

DAILY EXERCISE

Water Intake
# of 8 oz. glasses
◯◯◯
◯◯◯
◯◯◯

ENERGY LEVEL:
◯ low
◯ medium
◯ high

Activity	Hrs./Mins.	Cal. Burned
DAILY TOTALS:		

CALORIE CALCULATOR

	−		=		−		=	
TOTAL CALORIE INTAKE		TOTAL CALORIES BURNED		NET CALORIES		BMR (Basal Metabolic Rate)		DAILY NET CALORIE GAIN OR LOSS

Day 3

DATE: _____ WEIGHT: _____

NUTRITIONAL INTAKE

FOOD/BEVERAGE	Qty.	Calories	Fat	Carbs	Other
_____	_____				
_____	_____				
_____	_____				
_____	_____				
_____	_____				
_____	_____				
_____	_____				
_____	_____				
_____	_____				
_____	_____				
_____	_____				
DAILY INTAKE TOTALS:					

DAILY EXERCISE

☑ **Water Intake**
# of 8 oz. glasses

◯◯◯
◯◯◯
◯◯◯

ENERGY LEVEL:

◯ low

◯ medium

◯ high

Activity	Hrs./Mins.	Cal. Burned
_____		
_____		
_____		
_____		
_____		
DAILY TOTALS:		

CALORIE CALCULATOR

	−		=		−		=	
TOTAL CALORIE INTAKE		TOTAL CALORIES BURNED		NET CALORIES		BMR (Basal Metabolic Rate)		DAILY NET CALORIE GAIN OR LOSS

Day 4

DATE: _____ WEIGHT: _____

NUTRITIONAL INTAKE

FOOD/BEVERAGE	Qty.	Calories	Fat	Carbs	Other
DAILY INTAKE TOTALS:					

DAILY EXERCISE

Water Intake
of 8 oz. glasses

◯◯◯
◯◯◯
◯◯◯

ERGY LEVEL:

◯ low
◯ medium
◯ high

Activity	Hrs./Mins.	Cal. Burned
DAILY TOTALS:		

CALORIE CALCULATOR

	−		=		−		=	
AL CALORIE INTAKE		TOTAL CALORIES BURNED		NET CALORIES		BMR (Basal Metabolic Rate)		DAILY NET CALORIE GAIN OR LOSS

Day 5

DATE: _____   WEIGHT: _____

NUTRITIONAL INTAKE

⬤ FOOD/BEVERAGE	Qty.	Calories	Fat	Carbs	Other
_____	_____				
_____	_____				
_____	_____				
_____	_____				
_____	_____				
_____	_____				
_____	_____				
_____	_____				
_____	_____				
_____	_____				
DAILY INTAKE TOTALS:					

DAILY EXERCISE

☑ **Water Intake**
# of 8 oz. glasses

◯◯◯
◯◯◯
◯◯◯

ENERGY LEVEL:

◯ low
◯ medium
◯ high

Activity	Hrs./Mins.	Cal. Burned
_____	_____	
_____	_____	
_____	_____	
_____	_____	
_____	_____	
DAILY TOTALS:		

CALORIE CALCULATOR

☐	−	☐	=	☐	−	☐	=	☐
TOTAL CALORIE INTAKE		TOTAL CALORIES BURNED		NET CALORIES		BMR (Basal Metabolic Rate)		DAILY NET CALO GAIN OR LO

DATE: _____ WEIGHT: _____

NUTRITIONAL INTAKE

FOOD/BEVERAGE	Qty.	Calories	Fat	Carbs	Other
_____	_____				
_____	_____				
_____	_____				
_____	_____				
_____	_____				
_____	_____				
_____	_____				
_____	_____				
_____	_____				
_____	_____				
_____	_____				
DAILY INTAKE TOTALS:					

DAILY EXERCISE

☑ Water Intake
# of 8 oz. glasses

◯◯◯
◯◯◯
◯◯◯

ENERGY LEVEL:
◯ low
◯ medium
◯ high

Activity	Hrs./Mins.	Cal. Burned
_____		
_____		
_____		
_____		
_____		
DAILY TOTALS:		

CALORIE CALCULATOR

	−		=		−		=	
TOTAL CALORIE INTAKE		TOTAL CALORIES BURNED		NET CALORIES		BMR (Basal Metabolic Rate)		DAILY NET CALORIE GAIN OR LOSS

Day 7

DATE: _____ WEIGHT: _____

NUTRITIONAL INTAKE

FOOD/BEVERAGE	Qty.	Calories	Fat	Carbs	Other
DAILY INTAKE TOTALS:					

DAILY EXERCISE

☑ **Water Intake**
# of 8 oz. glasses

◯◯◯
◯◯◯
◯◯◯

ENERGY LEVEL:

◯ low

◯ medium

◯ high

Activity	Hrs./Mins.	Cal. Burned
DAILY TOTALS:		

CALORIE CALCULATOR

	−		=		−		=	
TOTAL CALORIE INTAKE		TOTAL CALORIES BURNED		NET CALORIES		BMR (Basal Metabolic Rate)		DAILY NET CALORIE GAIN OR LOSS

208 SEXY ABS DIET POCKET GUIDE

Day 8

NUTRITIONAL INTAKE

FOOD/BEVERAGE	Qty.	Calories	Fat	Carbs	Other
DAILY INTAKE TOTALS:					

DAILY EXERCISE

Water Intake
# of 8 oz. glasses

☐☐☐
☐☐☐
☐☐☐

ENERGY LEVEL:
☐ low
☐ medium
☐ high

Activity	Hrs./Mins.	Cal. Burned
DAILY TOTALS:		

CALORIE CALCULATOR

TOTAL CALORIE INTAKE	−	TOTAL CALORIES BURNED	=	NET CALORIES	−	BMR (Basal Metabolic Rate)	=	DAILY NET CALORIE GAIN OR LOSS

Day 9

DATE: _____ WEIGHT: _____

NUTRITIONAL INTAKE

FOOD/BEVERAGE	Qty.	Calories	Fat	Carbs	Other
_____	_____				
_____	_____				
_____	_____				
_____	_____				
_____	_____				
_____	_____				
_____	_____				
_____	_____				
_____	_____				
_____	_____				
_____	_____				
DAILY INTAKE TOTALS:					

DAILY EXERCISE

☑ **Water Intake**
# of 8 oz. glasses

◯◯◯
◯◯◯
◯◯◯

ENERGY LEVEL:

◯ low
◯ medium
◯ high

Activity	Hrs./Mins.	Cal. Burned
_____	_____	
_____	_____	
_____	_____	
_____	_____	
_____	_____	
DAILY TOTALS:		

CALORIE CALCULATOR

	−		=		−		=	
TOTAL CALORIE INTAKE		TOTAL CALORIES BURNED		NET CALORIES		BMR (Basal Metabolic Rate)		DAILY NET CALOR GAIN OR LOS

DATE: _____ WEIGHT: _____

NUTRITIONAL INTAKE

FOOD/BEVERAGE	Qty.	Calories	Fat	Carbs	Other
DAILY INTAKE TOTALS:					

DAILY EXERCISE

☑ **Water Intake**
# of 8 oz. glasses

◯◯◯
◯◯◯
◯◯◯

NERGY LEVEL:

◻ low
◻ medium
◻ high

Activity	Hrs./Mins.	Cal. Burned
	DAILY TOTALS:	

CALORIE CALCULATOR

	−		=		−		=	
TOTAL CALORIE INTAKE		TOTAL CALORIES BURNED		NET CALORIES		BMR (Basal Metabolic Rate)		DAILY NET CALORIE GAIN OR LOSS

Day 11

DATE: _____ WEIGHT: _____

NUTRITIONAL INTAKE

🍎 FOOD/BEVERAGE	Qty.	Calories	Fat	Carbs	Other
_____	_____				
_____	_____				
_____	_____				
_____	_____				
_____	_____				
_____	_____				
_____	_____				
_____	_____				
_____	_____				
_____	_____				
_____	_____				
DAILY INTAKE TOTALS:					

DAILY EXERCISE

☑ Water Intake # of 8 oz. glasses	Activity	Hrs./Mins.	Cal. Burned
◯◯◯	_____	_____	
◯◯◯	_____	_____	
◯◯◯	_____	_____	
ENERGY LEVEL:	_____	_____	
◯ low	_____	_____	
◯ medium			
◯ high	**DAILY TOTALS:**		

CALORIE CALCULATOR

	−		=		−		=	
TOTAL CALORIE INTAKE		TOTAL CALORIES BURNED		NET CALORIES		BMR (Basal Metabolic Rate)		DAILY NET CALORIE GAIN OR LOSS

Day 12

DATE: _____ WEIGHT: _____

NUTRITIONAL INTAKE

FOOD/BEVERAGE	Qty.	Calories	Fat	Carbs	Other
DAILY INTAKE TOTALS:					

DAILY EXERCISE

Water Intake
# of 8 oz. glasses

◯◯◯
◯◯◯
◯◯◯

NERGY LEVEL:

◯ low
◯ medium
◯ high

Activity	Hrs./Mins.	Cal. Burned
DAILY TOTALS:		

CALORIE CALCULATOR

	−		=		−		=	
TOTAL CALORIE INTAKE		TOTAL CALORIES BURNED		NET CALORIES		BMR (Basal Metabolic Rate)		DAILY NET CALORIE GAIN OR LOSS

Day 13

DATE: _____ WEIGHT: _____

NUTRITIONAL INTAKE

FOOD/BEVERAGE	Qty.	Calories	Fat	Carbs	Other
_____	_____				
_____	_____				
_____	_____				
_____	_____				
_____	_____				
_____	_____				
_____	_____				
_____	_____				
_____	_____				
_____	_____				
DAILY INTAKE TOTALS:					

DAILY EXERCISE

☑ **Water Intake**
# of 8 oz. glasses

▢▢▢
▢▢▢
▢▢▢

ENERGY LEVEL:

▢ low
▢ medium
▢ high

Activity	Hrs./Mins.	Cal. Burned
_____	_____	
_____	_____	
_____	_____	
_____	_____	
_____	_____	
DAILY TOTALS:		

CALORIE CALCULATOR

	−		=		−		=	
TOTAL CALORIE INTAKE		TOTAL CALORIES BURNED		NET CALORIES		BMR (Basal Metabolic Rate)		DAILY NET CALORIE GAIN OR LOSS

Day 14

DATE: _____ WEIGHT: _____

NUTRITIONAL INTAKE

FOOD/BEVERAGE	Qty.	Calories	Fat	Carbs	Other
_____	_____				
_____	_____				
_____	_____				
_____	_____				
_____	_____				
_____	_____				
_____	_____				
_____	_____				
_____	_____				
_____	_____				
_____	_____				
DAILY INTAKE TOTALS:					

DAILY EXERCISE

☑ **Water Intake**
# of 8 oz. glasses

◯◯◯
◯◯◯
◯◯◯

ENERGY LEVEL:

◯ low
◯ medium
◯ high

Activity	Hrs./Mins.	Cal. Burned
_____	_____	
_____	_____	
_____	_____	
_____	_____	
_____	_____	
_____	_____	
DAILY TOTALS:		

CALORIE CALCULATOR

	−		=		−		=	
TOTAL CALORIE INTAKE		TOTAL CALORIES BURNED		NET CALORIES		BMR (Basal Metabolic Rate)		DAILY NET CALORIE GAIN OR LOSS

Day 15

DATE: _____ WEIGHT: _____

NUTRITIONAL INTAKE

FOOD/BEVERAGE	Qty.	Calories	Fat	Carbs	Other
_____	_____				
_____	_____				
_____	_____				
_____	_____				
_____	_____				
_____	_____				
_____	_____				
_____	_____				
_____	_____				
_____	_____				
_____	_____				
_____	_____				
DAILY INTAKE TOTALS:					

DAILY EXERCISE

☑ **Water Intake**
# of 8 oz. glasses

◯◯◯
◯◯◯
◯◯◯

ENERGY LEVEL:

◯ low
◯ medium
◯ high

Activity	Hrs./Mins.	Cal. Burned
_____	_____	
_____	_____	
_____	_____	
_____	_____	
_____	_____	
DAILY TOTALS:		

CALORIE CALCULATOR

	–		=		–		=	
TOTAL CALORIE INTAKE		TOTAL CALORIES BURNED		NET CALORIES		BMR (Basal Metabolic Rate)		DAILY NET CALORIE GAIN OR LOSS

Day 16

DATE: _____ WEIGHT: _____

NUTRITIONAL INTAKE

FOOD/BEVERAGE	Qty.	Calories	Fat	Carbs	Other
_____	_____				
_____	_____				
_____	_____				
_____	_____				
_____	_____				
_____	_____				
_____	_____				
_____	_____				
_____	_____				
_____	_____				
DAILY INTAKE TOTALS:					

DAILY EXERCISE

☑ Water Intake
# of 8 oz. glasses

◯◯◯
◯◯◯
◯◯◯

ENERGY LEVEL:

◯ low
◯ medium
◯ high

Activity	Hrs./Mins.	Cal. Burned
_____	_____	
_____	_____	
_____	_____	
_____	_____	
_____	_____	
DAILY TOTALS:		

CALORIE CALCULATOR

	−		=		−		=	
TOTAL CALORIE INTAKE		TOTAL CALORIES BURNED		NET CALORIES		BMR (Basal Metabolic Rate)		DAILY NET CALORIE GAIN OR LOSS

Day 17

NUTRITIONAL INTAKE

FOOD/BEVERAGE	Qty.	Calories	Fat	Carbs	Other
_____	_____				
_____	_____				
_____	_____				
_____	_____				
_____	_____				
_____	_____				
_____	_____				
_____	_____				
_____	_____				
_____	_____				
_____	_____				
DAILY INTAKE TOTALS:					

DAILY EXERCISE

☑ **Water Intake**
# of 8 oz. glasses

☐☐☐
☐☐☐
☐☐☐

ENERGY LEVEL:

☐ low
☐ medium
☐ high

Activity	Hrs./Mins.	Cal. Burned
_____	_____	
_____	_____	
_____	_____	
_____	_____	
_____	_____	
DAILY TOTALS:		

CALORIE CALCULATOR

	−		=		−		=	
TOTAL CALORIE INTAKE		TOTAL CALORIES BURNED		NET CALORIES		BMR (Basal Metabolic Rate)		DAILY NET CALORIE GAIN OR LOSS

DATE: _____ WEIGHT: _____

NUTRITIONAL INTAKE

FOOD/BEVERAGE	Qty.	Calories	Fat	Carbs	Other
DAILY INTAKE TOTALS:					

DAILY EXERCISE

Water Intake
# of 8 oz. glasses

ENERGY LEVEL:
- [ ] low
- [ ] medium
- [ ] high

Activity	Hrs./Mins.	Cal. Burned
DAILY TOTALS:		

CALORIE CALCULATOR

	−		=		−		=	
TOTAL CALORIE INTAKE		TOTAL CALORIES BURNED		NET CALORIES		BMR (Basal Metabolic Rate)		DAILY NET CALORIE GAIN OR LOSS

Day 19

DATE: _____ WEIGHT: _____

NUTRITIONAL INTAKE

FOOD/BEVERAGE	Qty.	Calories	Fat	Carbs	Other
_____	_____				
_____	_____				
_____	_____				
_____	_____				
_____	_____				
_____	_____				
_____	_____				
_____	_____				
_____	_____				
_____	_____				
DAILY INTAKE TOTALS:					

DAILY EXERCISE

☑ **Water Intake**
# of 8 oz. glasses

◯◯◯
◯◯◯
◯◯◯

ENERGY LEVEL:

◯ low
◯ medium
◯ high

Activity	Hrs./Mins.	Cal. Burned
_____	_____	
_____	_____	
_____	_____	
_____	_____	
_____	_____	
DAILY TOTALS:		

CALORIE CALCULATOR

	−		=		−		=	
TOTAL CALORIE INTAKE		TOTAL CALORIES BURNED		NET CALORIES		BMR (Basal Metabolic Rate)		DAILY NET CALORIE GAIN OR LOSS

220 SEXY ABS DIET POCKET GUIDE

DATE: _____ WEIGHT: _____

NUTRITIONAL INTAKE

FOOD/BEVERAGE	Qty.	Calories	Fat	Carbs	Other
DAILY INTAKE TOTALS:					

DAILY EXERCISE

Water Intake
of 8 oz. glasses

◯◯◯
◯◯◯
◯◯◯

ENERGY LEVEL:

◯ low
◯ medium
◯ high

Activity	Hrs./Mins.	Cal. Burned
DAILY TOTALS:		

CALORIE CALCULATOR

	−		=		−		=	
TOTAL CALORIE INTAKE		TOTAL CALORIES BURNED		NET CALORIES		BMR (Basal Metabolic Rate)		DAILY NET CALORIE GAIN OR LOSS

Day 21   DATE: _____   WEIGHT: _____

NUTRITIONAL INTAKE

FOOD/BEVERAGE	Qty.	Calories	Fat	Carbs	Other
_____	_____				
_____	_____				
_____	_____				
_____	_____				
_____	_____				
_____	_____				
_____	_____				
_____	_____				
_____	_____				
_____	_____				
DAILY INTAKE TOTALS:					

DAILY EXERCISE

	Activity	Hrs./Mins.	Cal. Burne
☑ **Water Intake** # of 8 oz. glasses			

☐☐☐
☐☐☐
☐☐☐

	Activity	Hrs./Mins.	Cal. Burne
	_____	_____	
	_____	_____	
	_____	_____	

ENERGY LEVEL:

☐ low
☐ medium
☐ high

DAILY TOTALS:

CALORIE CALCULATOR

	−		=		−		=	

TOTAL CALORIE INTAKE − TOTAL CALORIES BURNED = NET CALORIES − BMR (Basal Metabolic Rate) = DAILY NET CALO GAIN OR LO

Day 22

DATE: _____   WEIGHT: _____

NUTRITIONAL INTAKE

FOOD/BEVERAGE	Qty.	Calories	Fat	Carbs	Other
DAILY INTAKE TOTALS:					

DAILY EXERCISE

☑ **Water Intake**
# of 8 oz. glasses

◯◯◯
◯◯◯
◯◯◯

ENERGY LEVEL:

◯ low
◯ medium
◯ high

Activity	Hrs./Mins.	Cal. Burned
DAILY TOTALS:		

CALORIE CALCULATOR

	−		=		−		=	
TOTAL CALORIE INTAKE		TOTAL CALORIES BURNED		NET CALORIES		BMR (Basal Metabolic Rate)		DAILY NET CALORIE GAIN OR LOSS

Day 23

NUTRITIONAL INTAKE

FOOD/BEVERAGE	Qty.	Calories	Fat	Carbs	Other
DAILY INTAKE TOTALS:					

DAILY EXERCISE

☑ Water Intake
# of 8 oz. glasses

☐☐☐
☐☐☐
☐☐☐

ENERGY LEVEL:

☐ low

☐ medium

☐ high

Activity	Hrs./Mins.	Cal. Burned
	DAILY TOTALS:	

CALORIE CALCULATOR

	−	=	−	=
TOTAL CALORIE INTAKE	TOTAL CALORIES BURNED	NET CALORIES	BMR (Basal Metabolic Rate)	DAILY NET CALORIE GAIN OR LOSS

Day 24

DATE: _____ WEIGHT: _____

NUTRITIONAL INTAKE

FOOD/BEVERAGE	Qty.	Calories	Fat	Carbs	Other
DAILY INTAKE TOTALS:					

DAILY EXERCISE

☑ **Water Intake**
# of 8 oz. glasses

◯◯◯
◯◯◯
◯◯◯

ENERGY LEVEL:

◯ low
◯ medium
◯ high

Activity	Hrs./Mins.	Cal. Burned
DAILY TOTALS:		

CALORIE CALCULATOR

	−		=		−		=	
TOTAL CALORIE INTAKE		TOTAL CALORIES BURNED		NET CALORIES		BMR (Basal Metabolic Rate)		DAILY NET CALORIE GAIN OR LOSS

Day 25

DATE: _____ WEIGHT: _____

NUTRITIONAL INTAKE

FOOD/BEVERAGE	Qty.	Calories	Fat	Carbs	Other
_____	_____				
_____	_____				
_____	_____				
_____	_____				
_____	_____				
_____	_____				
_____	_____				
_____	_____				
_____	_____				
_____	_____				
DAILY INTAKE TOTALS:					

DAILY EXERCISE

☑ **Water Intake**
# of 8 oz. glasses

☐☐☐
☐☐☐
☐☐☐

ENERGY LEVEL:

☐ low
☐ medium
☐ high

Activity	Hrs./Mins.	Cal. Burned
_____	_____	
_____	_____	
_____	_____	
_____	_____	
_____	_____	
DAILY TOTALS:		

CALORIE CALCULATOR

	−		=		−		=	
TOTAL CALORIE INTAKE		TOTAL CALORIES BURNED		NET CALORIES		BMR (Basal Metabolic Rate)		DAILY NET CALOR GAIN OR LOS

DATE: _____ WEIGHT: _____

NUTRITIONAL INTAKE

FOOD/BEVERAGE	Qty.	Calories	Fat	Carbs	Other
DAILY INTAKE TOTALS:					

DAILY EXERCISE

☑ **Water Intake**
# of 8 oz. glasses

◯◯◯
◯◯◯
◯◯◯

NERGY LEVEL:

◯ low
◯ medium
◯ high

Activity	Hrs./Mins.	Cal. Burned
DAILY TOTALS:		

CALORIE CALCULATOR

	−		=		−		=	
OTAL CALORIE INTAKE		TOTAL CALORIES BURNED		NET CALORIES		BMR (Basal Metabolic Rate)		DAILY NET CALORIE GAIN OR LOSS

Day 27   DATE: _____ WEIGHT: _____

NUTRITIONAL INTAKE

🍎 FOOD/BEVERAGE	Qty.	Calories	Fat	Carbs	Other
_____	_____				
_____	_____				
_____	_____				
_____	_____				
_____	_____				
_____	_____				
_____	_____				
_____	_____				
_____	_____				
_____	_____				
_____	_____				
_____	_____				
DAILY INTAKE TOTALS:					

DAILY EXERCISE

☑ **Water Intake**
# of 8 oz. glasses

◯◯◯
◯◯◯
◯◯◯

ENERGY LEVEL:

◯ low

◯ medium

◯ high

Activity	Hrs./Mins.	Cal. Burned
_____	_____	
_____	_____	
_____	_____	
_____	_____	
_____	_____	
DAILY TOTALS:		

CALORIE CALCULATOR

	−		=		−		=	
TOTAL CALORIE INTAKE		TOTAL CALORIES BURNED		NET CALORIES		BMR (Basal Metabolic Rate)		DAILY NET CALORIE GAIN OR LOSS

Day 28

DATE: _____ WEIGHT: _____

NUTRITIONAL INTAKE

FOOD/BEVERAGE	Qty.	Calories	Fat	Carbs	Other
_____	_____				
_____	_____				
_____	_____				
_____	_____				
_____	_____				
_____	_____				
_____	_____				
_____	_____				
_____	_____				
_____	_____				
_____	_____				
DAILY INTAKE TOTALS:					

DAILY EXERCISE

☑ **Water Intake**
# of 8 oz. glasses

Activity	Hrs./Mins.	Cal. Burned
_____	_____	
_____	_____	
_____	_____	
_____	_____	
_____	_____	

NERGY LEVEL:

☐ low
☐ medium
☐ high

DAILY TOTALS:

CALORIE CALCULATOR

[____]	−	[____]	=	[____]	−	[____]	=	[____]
TOTAL CALORIE INTAKE		TOTAL CALORIES BURNED		NET CALORIES		BMR (Basal Metabolic Rate)		DAILY NET CALORIE GAIN OR LOSS

Day 29

DATE: _____ WEIGHT: _____

NUTRITIONAL INTAKE

FOOD/BEVERAGE	Qty.	Calories	Fat	Carbs	Other
DAILY INTAKE TOTALS:					

DAILY EXERCISE

Activity	Hrs./Mins.	Cal. Burned

☑ **Water Intake**
# of 8 oz. glasses

◯◯◯
◯◯◯
◯◯◯

ENERGY LEVEL:

◯ low

◯ medium

◯ high

DAILY TOTALS:

CALORIE CALCULATOR

TOTAL CALORIE INTAKE	−	TOTAL CALORIES BURNED	=	NET CALORIES	−	BMR (Basal Metabolic Rate)	=	DAILY NET CALORIE GAIN OR LOSS

NUTRITIONAL INTAKE

FOOD/BEVERAGE	Qty.	Calories	Fat	Carbs	Other
DAILY INTAKE TOTALS:					

DAILY EXERCISE

☑ **Water Intake**
# of 8 oz. glasses

◯◯◯
◯◯◯
◯◯◯

ENERGY LEVEL:
☐ low
☐ medium
☐ high

Activity	Hrs./Mins.	Cal. Burned
DAILY TOTALS:		

CALORIE CALCULATOR

TOTAL CALORIE INTAKE	−	TOTAL CALORIES BURNED	=	NET CALORIES	−	BMR (Basal Metabolic Rate)	=	DAILY NET CALORIE GAIN OR LOSS

Tell Us Your Weight-Loss Success Story!

We love hearing about our readers' weight-loss success stories!

Please tell us your story, your initial weight and measurements, your expectations for this diet and fitness program, etc. Tell us what you liked or didn't like about this book, and what you found useful or wished we had included. Tell us how difficult or how easy it was for you to stick to your diet or maintain the exercise program. Now, tell us how you feel with your new slimmer and healthier body. Share your advice for others who are struggling with their weight.

Please include the following information:

- Your name:
- Phone number:
- E-mail:
- Your story!
- Before and After photos, if possible

Please email this information to:
info@WSPublishingGroup.com
Or send a letter to:

WS Publishing Group
15373 Innovation Drive, Suite 360
San Diego, CA 92128.

Notes:

Notes:

_____

_____

_____

_____

_____

_____

_____

_____

_____

_____

_____

_____

_____

_____

_____

_____

_____

_____

_____

_____

Notes:

Interval Timer
Workout & Fitness PRO

Working out has never been easier!
The *Interval Timer: Workout & Fitness PRO* keeps you motivated and makes exercise fun.

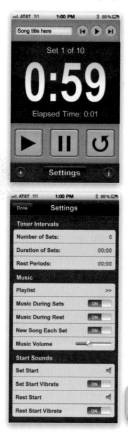

Special Features:

- Large, easy-to-read display & buttons
- Tracks number of sets performed
- Shows elapsed time and rest period
- Gives multiple cue options for sets and rest periods
- Plays music from your iTunes library

So easy to use:

1) Enter the number of sets you desire, well as the length of time for each set a rest period.

2) Select a custom ringtone or set your iPhone to vibrate to cue you at the start of each set and/or rest period.

Or, play your favorite music from your iTunes Library. You can even choose a new song to start off each set!

Search the iTunes App store for Interval Timer Workout & Fitness PRO